Confirmatory Factor Analysis

POCKET GUIDES TO
SOCIAL WORK RESEARCH METHODS

Series Editor
Tony Tripodi, DSW
Professor Emeritus, Ohio State University

Determining Sample Size
Balancing Power, Precision, and Practicality
Patrick Dattalo

Preparing Research Articles
Bruce A. Thyer

Systematic Reviews and Meta-Analysis
Julia H. Littell, Jacqueline Corcoran, and Vijayan Pillai

Historical Research
Elizabeth Ann Danto

Confirmatory Factor Analysis
Donna Harrington

DONNA HARRINGTON

Confirmatory Factor Analysis

OXFORD
UNIVERSITY PRESS

2009

OXFORD

UNIVERSITY PRESS

Oxford University Press, Inc., publishes works that further
Oxford University's objective of excellence
in research, scholarship, and education.

Oxford   New York
Auckland   Cape Town   Dar es Salaam   Hong Kong   Karachi
Kuala Lumpur   Madrid   Melbourne   Mexico City   Nairobi
New Delhi   Shanghai   Taipei   Toronto

With offices in
Argentina   Austria   Brazil   Chile   Czech Republic   France   Greece
Guatemala   Hungary   Italy   Japan   Poland   Portugal   Singapore
South Korea   Switzerland   Thailand   Turkey   Ukraine   Vietnam

Published by Oxford University Press, Inc.
198 Madison Avenue, New York, New York 10016

www.oup.com

Oxford is a registered trademark of Oxford University Press

Library of Congress Cataloging-in-Publication Data
Harrington, Donna. Confirmatory factor analysis / Donna Harrington.
p. cm.
Includes bibliographical references and index.
ISBN 978-0-19-533988-8
1. Social service—Research.   2. Evaluation research (Social action programs)
3. Evidence-based social work.   I. Title.
HV11.H5576 2009 361.0072—dc22

1   3   5   7   9   8   6   4   2

Printed in the United States of America
on acid-free paper

To my parents,
Pauline and Robert Harrington

And to my grandmother,
Marguerite A. Burke

Acknowledgments

I am incredibly grateful to several people for their guidance, encouragement, and constructive feedback. I would like to thank Dr. Joan Levy Zlotnik, Executive Director of the Institute for the Advancement of Social Work Research (IASWR) for inviting me to do a workshop on confirmatory factor analysis (CFA). Much of the approach and several of the examples used here were developed for that two-day workshop; the workshop participants were enthusiastic and well prepared, and this book builds on the questions they asked and the feedback they provided. Dr. Elizabeth Greeno helped plan and co-led the workshop; one of her articles is used as a CFA example in this book. This book would not exist if Dr. Tony Tripodi, the series editor for these pocket books, had not seen the IASWR workshop announcement and invited me to do a book proposal; his comments and suggests on the outline of the book were very helpful. The reviewers of the book proposal and draft of this book were wonderful and I greatly appreciate all their feedback. I have also been very lucky to work with Maura Roessner and Mallory Jensen at Oxford University Press, who have provided guidance throughout this process.

I also have to thank the graduates and students of the University of Maryland social work doctoral program over the past 14 years—they have taught me more about social work, statistics, and teaching than I can ever hope to pass on to anyone else. One doctoral student in particular, Ms. Ann LeFevre, has been unbelievably helpful—she found examples of CFA in the social work literature, followed the Amos instructions to see if you could actually complete a CFA with only this book for guidance, and read several drafts, always providing helpful suggestions and comments about how to make the material as accessible as possible for readers. Finally, I have to thank my husband, Ken Brawn, for technical assistance with the computer files, and more importantly, all the meals he fixed while I was working on this.

Contents

1   Introduction   3

2   Creating a Confirmatory Factor Analysis Model   21

3   Requirements for Conducting Confirmatory Factor Analysis:
    Data Considerations   36

4   Assessing Confirmatory Factor Analysis Model Fit and
    Model Revision   50

5   Use of Confirmatory Factor Analysis with Multiple Groups   78

6   Other Issues   100

    Glossary   105

    Appendix A: Brief Introduction to Using Amos   107

    References   115

    Index   121

Confirmatory Factor Analysis

1

Introduction

This pocket guide will cover *confirmatory factor analysis* (CFA), which is used for four major purposes: *(1)* psychometric evaluation of measures; *(2)* construct validation; *(3)* testing method effects; and *(4)* testing measurement invariance (e.g., across groups or populations) (Brown, 2006). This book is intended for readers who are new to CFA and are interested in developing an understanding of this methodology so they can more effectively read and critique research that uses CFA methods. In addition, it is hoped that this book will serve as a nontechnical introduction to this topic for readers who plan to use CFA but who want a nonmathematical, conceptual, applied introduction to CFA before turning to the more specialized literature on this topic. To make this book as applied as possible, we will take two small data sets and develop detailed examples of CFA analyses; the data will be available on the Internet so readers can replicate analyses as they work through the book. A brief glossary of some common CFA terms is provided. Finally, the programs for running the sample analyses in Amos 7.0 are included in this book, and very brief instructions for using the software are provided in Appendix A. However, in general, this book is not intended as a guide to using the software, so information of this type is kept to a minimum.

When software instructions are presented, I have tried to select features and commands that seem unlikely to change in the near future.

A word of caution: In attempting to provide a conceptual understanding of CFA, there are times when I have used analogies, which I hope help illustrate the concepts. However, the analogies only work to a point and should not be taken literally. Also, in providing a nontechnical discussion, some details or finer points will be lost. It is hoped that interested readers—especially those planning to use CFA on their own data—will turn to some of the more technical resources provided at the end of each chapter for more information.

This chapter focuses on what CFA is, when to use it, and how it compares to other common data analysis techniques, including principal components analysis (PCA), exploratory factor analysis (EFA), and structural equation modeling (SEM). This is a brief discussion, with references to other publications for more detail on the other techniques. The social work literature includes a number of good examples of the use of CFA, and a few of these articles are briefly summarized to illustrate how CFA can be used. *Research on Social Work Practice* publishes numerous articles that examine the validity of social work assessments and measures; several of these articles use CFA and are cited as examples in this book.

Significance of Confirmatory Factor Analysis for Social Work Research

Social work researchers need to have measures with good reliability and validity that are appropriate for use across diverse populations. Development of psychometrically sound measures is an expensive and time-consuming process, and CFA may be one step in the development process. Because researchers often do not have the time or the resources to develop a new measure, they may need to use existing measures. In addition to savings in time and costs, using existing measures also helps to make research findings comparable across studies when the same measure is used in more than one study. However, when using an existing measure, it is important to examine whether the measure is appropriate for the population included in the current study. In these circumstances, CFA can be used to examine whether the original structure of the measure works well in the new population.

Uses of Confirmatory Factor Analysis

Within social work, CFA can be used for multiple purposes, including—but not limited to—the development of new measures, evaluation of the psychometric properties of new and existing measures, and examination of method effects. CFA can also be used to examine construct validation and whether a measure is invariant or unchanging across groups, populations, or time. It is important to note that these uses are overlapping rather than truly distinct, and unfortunately there is a lack of consistency in how several of the terms related to construct validity are used in the social work literature. Several of these uses are briefly discussed, and a number of examples from the social work literature are presented later in this chapter.

Development of New Measures and Construct Validation

Within the social work literature, there is often confusion and inconsistency about the different types and subtypes of validity. A full discussion of this issue is beyond the scope of this book, but a very brief discussion is provided for context so readers can see how CFA can be used to test specific aspects of validity. Construct validity in the broadest sense examines the relationships among the constructs. Constructs are unobserved and theoretical (e.g., factors or latent variables). However, although they are unobserved, there is often related theory that describes how constructs should be related to each other. According to Cronbach and Meehl (1955), construct validity refers to an examination of a measure of an attribute (or construct) that is not operationally defined or measured directly. During the process of establishing construct validity, the researcher tests specific hypotheses about how the measure is related to other measures based on theory.

Koeske (1994) distinguishes between two general validity concerns—specifically, the validity of conclusions and the validity of measures. Conclusion validity focuses on the validity of the interpretation of study findings and includes four subtypes of validity: internal, external, statistical conclusion, and experimental construct (for more information, see Koeske, 1994 or Shaddish, Cook, & Campbell, 2002). Issues of conclusion validity go beyond what one can establish with CFA (or any other) statistical analysis. On the other hand, the validity of measures can be addressed, at least partially, through statistical analysis, and CFA can be one method for assessing aspects of the validity of measures.

Within measurement validity, there are three types: content, criterion, and construct validity; within construct validity, there are three subtypes: convergent, discriminant, and theoretical (or nomological) validity (Koeske, 1994). Discriminant validity is demonstrated when measures of different concepts or constructs are distinct (i.e., there are low correlations among the concepts) (Bagozzi, Yi, & Phillips, 1991). Although the criteria for what counts as a low correlation vary across sources, Brown (2006) notes that correlations between constructs of 0.85 or above indicate poor discriminant validity. When measures of the same concept are highly correlated, there is evidence of convergent validity (Bagozzi et al., 1991); however, it is important to note that the measures must use different methods (e.g., self-report and observation) to avoid problems of shared-method variance when establishing convergent validity (Koeske, 1994). For example, if we are interested in job satisfaction, we may look for a strong relationship between self-reported job satisfaction and co-workers' ratings of an employee's level of job satisfaction. If we find this pattern of relationships, then we have evidence of convergent validity. If we believe that job satisfaction and general life satisfaction are two distinct constructs, then there should be a low correlation between them, which would demonstrate discriminant validity.

When examining construct validity, it is important to note that the same correlation between two latent variables could be good or bad, depending on the relationship expected. If theory indicates that job satisfaction and burnout are separate constructs, then based on theory, we expect to find a low or moderate correlation between them. If we find a correlation of –0.36, then we have evidence of discriminant validity, as predicted by the theory. However, if we find a correlation of –0.87, then we do not have evidence of discriminant validity because the correlation is too high. If theory had suggested that job satisfaction and burnout are measuring the same construct, then we would be looking for convergent validity (assuming we have different methods of measuring these two constructs), and we would interpret a correlation of –0.36 as not supporting convergent validity because it is too low, but the correlation of –0.87 would suggest good convergent validity. The important thing to note here is that the underlying theory is the basis on which decisions about construct validity are built.

Within this broad discussion of construct validity, CFA has a limited, but important role. Specifically, CFA can be used to examine structural (or factorial) validity, such as whether a construct is unidimensional or multidimensional and how the constructs (and subconstructs) are interrelated. CFA can be used to examine the latent (i.e., the unobserved underlying construct) structure of an instrument during scale development. For example, if an instrument is designed to have 40 items, which are divided into four factors with 10 items each, then CFA can be used to test whether the items are related to the hypothesized latent variables as expected, which indicates structural (or factorial) construct validity (Koeske, 1994). If earlier work is available, CFA can be used to verify the pattern of factors and loadings that were found. CFA can also be used to determine how an instrument should be scored (e.g., whether one total score is appropriate or a set of subscale scores is more appropriate). Finally, CFA can be used to estimate scale reliability.

Testing Method Effects

Method effects refer to relationships among variables or items that result from the measurement approach used (e.g., self-report), which includes how the questions are asked and the type of response options available. More broadly speaking, method effects may also include response bias effects such as social desirability (Podsakoff, MacKenzie, Lee, & Podsakoff, 2003). Common method effects are a widespread problem in research and may create a correlation between two measures, making it difficult to determine whether an observed correlation is the result of a true relationship or the result of shared methods. Different methods (e.g., self-report vs. observation) or wording (e.g., positively vs. negatively worded items) may result in a lower than expected correlation between constructs or in the suggestion that there are two or more constructs when, in reality, there is only one. For example, when measures have negatively and positively worded items, data analysis may suggest that there are two factors when only one was expected based on theory.

The Rosenberg Self-Esteem Scale (SES) provides a good example of this problem. The Rosenberg SES includes a combination of positively and negatively worded items. Early exploratory factor analysis work consistently yielded two factors—one consisting of the positively worded items and usually labeled positive self-esteem and one consisting of the negatively worded items and usually labeled negative self-esteem. However, there was no strong conceptual basis for the two-factor solution and further CFA research found that a one-factor model allowing for correlated residuals (i.e., method effects) provided a better fitting model than the earlier two-factor models (Brown, 2006). The conceptualization of the concept of self-esteem (i.e., the underlying theory) was a critical component of testing the one-factor solution with method effects. Method effects can exist in any measure, and one of the advantages of CFA is that it can be used to test for these effects, whereas some other types of data analysis cannot.

Testing Measurement Invariance Across Groups or Populations

Measurement invariance refers to testing how well models generalize across groups or time (Brown, 2006). This can be particularly important when testing whether a measure is appropriate for use in a population that is different from that with which the measure was developed and/or used with in the past. Multiple-group CFA can be used to test for measurement invariance and is discussed in detail in Chapter 5.

Comparison of Confirmatory Factor Analysis
With Other Data Analysis Techniques

Confirmatory factor analysis is strongly related to three other common data analysis techniques: EFA, PCA, and SEM. Although there are some similarities among these analyses, there are also some important distinctions that will be discussed below.

Before we begin discussing the data analysis techniques, we need to define a few terms that will be used throughout this section and the rest of this book (see also the Glossary for these and other terms used in this book). *Observed variables* are exactly what they sound like—bits of information that are actually observed, such as a person's response to a question, or a measured attribute, such as weight in pounds. Observed variables are also referred to as "indicators" or "items." *Latent variables* are unobserved (and are sometimes referred to as "unobserved variables" or "constructs"), but they are usually the things we are most interested in measuring. For example, research participants or clients can tell us if they have been feeling bothered, blue, or happy. Their self-report of how much they feel these things, such as their responses on the Center for Epidemiological Studies Depression Scale (Radloff, 1977), are observed variables. Depression, or the underlying construct, is a latent variable because we do not observe it directly; rather, we observe its symptoms.

Exploratory Factor Analysis

Exploratory factor analysis is used to identify the underlying factors or latent variables for a set of variables. The analysis accounts for the relationships (i.e., correlations, covariation, and variation) among the items (i.e., the observed variables or indicators). Exploratory factor analysis is based on the *common factor model*, where each observed variable is a linear function of one or more common factors (i.e., the underlying latent variables) and one unique factor (i.e., error- or item-specific information). It partitions item variance into two components: *(1)* Common variance, which is accounted for by underlying latent factors, and *(2)* unique variance, which is a combination of indicator-specific reliable variance and random error. Exploratory factor analysis is often considered a data-driven approach to identifying a smaller number of underlying factors or latent variables. It may also be used for generating basic explanatory theories and identifying the underlying latent variable structure; however, CFA testing or another approach to theory testing is needed to confirm the EFA findings (Haig, 2005).

Both EFA and CFA are based on the common factor model, so they are mathematically related procedures. EFA may be used as an exploratory first step during the development of a measure, and then CFA may be used as a second step to examine whether the structure identified in the EFA works in a new sample. In other words, CFA can be used to confirm the factor structure identified in the EFA. Unlike EFA, CFA requires pre-specification of all aspects of the model to be tested and is more theory-driven than data-driven. If a new measure is being developed with a very strong theoretical framework, then it may be possible to skip the initial EFA step and go directly to the CFA.

Principal Components Analysis

Principal components analysis is a data reduction technique used to identify a smaller number of underlying components in a set of observed variables or items. It accounts for the variance in the items, rather than the correlations among them. Unlike EFA and CFA, PCA is not based on the common factor model, and consequently, CFA may not work well when trying to replicate structures identified by PCA. There is debate about the use of PCA versus EFA. Stevens (2002) recommends PCA instead of EFA for several reasons, including the relatively simple mathematical model used in PCA and the lack of the factor indeterminacy problem found in factor analysis (i.e., factor analysis can yield an infinite number of sets of factor scores that are equally consistent with the same factor loadings, and there is no way to determine which set is the most accurate). However, others have argued that PCA should not be used in place of EFA (Brown, 2006). In practical applications with large samples and large numbers of items, PCA and EFA often yield similar results, although the loadings may be somewhat smaller in the EFA than the PCA.

For our purposes, it is most important to note that PCA may be used for similar purposes as EFA (e.g., data reduction), but it relies on a different mathematical model and therefore may not provide as firm a foundation for CFA as EFA. Finally, it is important to note that it is often difficult to tell from journal articles whether a PCA or an EFA was performed because authors often report doing a factor analysis but not what type of extraction they used (e.g., principal components, which results in a PCA, or some other form of extraction such as principal axis, which results in a factor analysis). Part of the difficulty may be the labeling used by popular software packages, such as SPSS, where principal components is the default form of extraction under the factor procedure.

As mentioned earlier, because EFA and CFA are both based on the common factor model, results from an EFA may be a stronger foundation for CFA than results from a PCA. Haig (2005) has suggested that EFA is "a latent variable method, thus distancing it from the data reduction method of principal components analysis. From this, it obviously follows that EFA should always be used in preference to principal components analysis when the underlying common causal structure of a domain is being investigated" (p. 321).

Structural Equation Modeling

Structural equation modeling is a general and broad family of analyses used to test measurement models (i.e., relationships among indicators and latent variables) and to examine the structural model of the relationships among latent variables. Structural equation modeling is widely used because it provides a quantitative method for testing substantive theories, and it explicitly accounts for measurement error, which is ever present in most disciplines (Raykov & Marcoulides, 2006), including social work. Structural equation modeling is a generic term that includes many common models that may include constructs that cannot be directly measured (i.e., latent variables) and potential errors of measurement (Raykov & Marcoulides, 2006).

A CFA model is sometimes described as a type of measurement model, and, as such, it is one type of analysis that falls under the SEM family. However, what distinguishes a CFA from a SEM model is that the CFA focuses on the relationships between the indicators and latent variables, whereas a SEM includes structural or causal paths between latent variables. CFA may be a stand-alone analysis or a component or preliminary step of a SEM analysis.

Software for Conducting Confirmatory Factor Analysis

There are several very good software packages for conducting confirmatory factor analyses, and all of them can be used to conduct CFA, SEM, and other analyses. Amos 7.0 (Arbuckle, 2006a) is used in this book. Although any of the major software packages would work well, Amos 7.0 was chosen because of its ease of use, particularly getting started with its graphics user interface[1]. Byrne (2001a) provides numerous examples using Amos software for conducting CFA and SEM analyses. Other software packages to consider include LISREL (see http://www.ssicentral.com/lisrel/index.html), Mplus (see http://www.statmodel.com/), EQS (see http://www.mvsoft.com/index.htm), or SAS CALIS (see http://v8doc.sas.com/sashtml/stat/chap19/sect1.htm). One other note—several of the software packages mentioned here have free demo versions that can be downloaded so you can try a software package before deciding whether to purchase it. Readers are encouraged to explore several of the major packages and think about how they want to use the software[2] before selecting one to purchase.

---

[1] Many software packages allow users to either type commands (i.e., write syntax) or use a menu (e.g., point-and-click) or graphics (e.g., drawing) interface to create the model to be analyzed. Some software (e.g., SPSS and Amos) allow the user to more than one option.

[2] Some software packages have more options than others. For example, Mplus has extensive Monte Carlo capabilities that are useful in conducting sample size analyses for CFA (see Chapter 3 for more information).

As Kline (2005, p. 7) notes, there has been a "near revolution" in the user friendliness of SEM software, especially with the introduction of easy-to-use graphics editors like Amos 7.0 provides. This ease of use is wonderful for users who have a good understanding of the analysis they plan to conduct, but there are also potential problems with these easy-to-use programs because users can create complex models without really understanding the underlying concepts. "To beginners it may appear that all one has to do is draw the model on the screen and let the computer take care of everything else. However, the reality is that things often can and do go wrong in SEM. Specifically, beginners often quickly discover the analyses fail because of technical problems, including a computer system crash or a terminated program run with many error messages or uninterpretable output" (Kline, 2005, pp. 7–8). In the analysis examples provided later in this book, we use data that is far from perfect so we can discuss some of the issues that can arise when conducting a CFA on real data.

Confirmatory Factor Analysis Examples from the Social Work Literature

With a growing emphasis on evidence-based practice in social work, there is a need for valid and reliable assessments. Although many journals publish articles on the development and testing of measures, *Research on Social Work Practice* has a particular emphasis on this, and therefore publishes a number of very good examples of CFA work. We briefly review several articles as examples of how CFA is used in the social work literature, and then end with a longer discussion of the Professional Opinion Scale, which has been subjected to CFA testing in two independent samples (Abbott, 2003 and Greeno, Hughes, Hayward, & Parker, 2007).

Caregiver Role Identity Scale

In an example of CFA used in scale development, Siebert and Siebert (2005) examined the factor structure of the Caregiver Role Identity Scale in a sample of 751 members of the North Carolina Chapter of NASW. The sample was randomly split so that exploratory and confirmatory analyses could be conducted. A principal components analysis was initially conducted, which yielded two components. This was followed by an EFA using principal axis extraction with oblique rotation on the first half of the sample. The EFA yielded a two-factor solution, with five items on the first factor and four items on the second factor; the two factors were significantly correlated ($r = 0.47$; $p < 0.00001$). The CFA was conducted using LISREL 8.54 and maximum likelihood (ML) estimation (estimation methods are discussed in Chapter 2) with the second half of the sample. The CFA resulted in several modifications to the factor structure identified in the EFA. Specifically, one item was dropped, resulting in an eight-item scale, with four items on each of the two factors. In addition, two error covariances were added (brief definitions for this and other terms can be found in the Glossary). The changes resulted in a significant improvement in fit, and the final model fit the data well (Siebert & Siebert, 2005). (We discuss model fit in Chapter 4, but briefly for now, you can think of model fit in much the same way that you evaluate how clothing fits—poorly fitting garments need to be tailored before they can be worn or used.) Siebert and Siebert concluded that the two-factor structure identified in the EFA was supported by the CFA and that the findings were consistent with role identity theory.

Child Abuse Potential Inventory

In an example of a CFA used to test the appropriateness of a measure across cultures, Chan, Lam, Chun, and So (2006) conducted a CFA on the Child Abuse Potential (CAP) Inventory using a sample of 897 Chinese mothers in Hong Kong. The CAP Inventory, developed by Milner (1986, 1989, and cited in Chan et al., 2006), is a self-administered measure with 160 items; 77 items are included in the six-factor clinical abuse scale. The purpose of the Chan et al. (2006) paper was to "evaluate if the factorial structure of the original 77-item Abuse Scale of the CAP found by Milner (1986) can be confirmed with data collected from a group of Chinese mothers in Hong Kong" (p. 1007). The CFA was conducted using LISREL 8.54. The CFA supported the original six-factor structure; 66 of the 77 items had loadings greater than 0.30, and "the model fit reasonably well" (Chan et al., 2006, p. 1012). Chan et al. (2006) concluded that "Although the CAP Abuse Scale is relevant for use with Chinese mothers in Hong Kong, it is clear that it is not parsimonious enough" (p. 1014). The low loadings (below 0.30) for 11 of the 77 items suggest that it may be possible to drop these items, resulting in a shorter scale.

Neglect Scale

In another example of CFA used to examine the use of a measure across populations, Harrington, Zuravin, DePanfilis, Ting, and Dubowitz (2002) used CFA to verify a factor structure identified in earlier work. The Neglect Scale was developed by Straus, Kinard, and Williams (1995) as an easy-to-administer, retrospective self-report measure of child neglect. Straus and colleagues suggested that the "relative lack of research on neglect may be due to the absence of a brief yet valid measure that can be used in epidemiological research" (pp. 1–2). The scale was found to have high internal consistency reliability and moderate construct validity in their sample of college students, most of whom were Caucasian.

Harrington et al. (2002) used the Neglect Scale in two studies of child maltreatment in Baltimore and were concerned that the measure would not work as well in a low-income, predominantly African-American sample as it had in Straus and colleagues' original work. An initial CFA indicated that the factor structure identified by Straus and colleagues did not fit the Baltimore data well; using modification indices and an expert panel, an alternative factor structure was identified that fit the data better. The CFA indicated that the original factor structure of the Neglect Scale did not fit well in the Baltimore sample, and modifications were needed for use of this measure with a low-income, minority population. However, because the model involved several modifications, it needs further study and replication.

Professional Opinion Scale

The Professional Opinion Scale (POS) is discussed in detail because it is one of the few social work measures on which two CFA studies have been performed; we briefly review both studies to provide an example of how a scale may evolve through the use of CFA. The POS was developed "to provide a methodologically sound and convenient means for assessing degree of commitment to social work values" (Abbott, 2003, p. 641). The 200 initial POS items were designed to reflect the recent (then-1980s) NASW policy statement topics, including AIDS, homelessness, domestic violence, substance abuse, human rights, and others. A panel of experts reviewed the items and retained 121 items determined to be clear and accurate and likely to be able to detect variability. Approximately half the items were worded negatively and half were worded positively. Positively worded items were reverse coded, and all items were coded as follows: 1= *strongly disagree*, 2 = *disagree*, 3 = *neutral*, 4 = *agree*, and 5 = *strongly agree*.

The initial subscale structure was identified using a diverse sample of 508 participants with data collected in 1988 (Abbott, 2003). Abbott (2003) refers to the data analysis as an EFA, but then states "The responses of the 1988 sample to the entire 121 POS items were examined using principal components factor analysis [with varimax rotation] . . . for the purpose of identifying value dimensions (factors) within the POS" (p. 647). Based on this analysis, "The 10 items having the highest loadings on each of the four remaining factors were retained, resulting in a 40-item, four-factor scale" (Abbott, 2003, p. 647). The labels for the four factors or value dimensions—"respect for basic rights, support of self-determination, sense of social responsibility, and commitment to individual freedom"— were based on the NASW Code of Ethics and the values identified in the social work literature (Abbott, 2003, p. 647). Finally, "A second analysis of the 1988 sample was conducted using maximum likelihood with oblique rotation with only the 40 items that make up the four factors" (Abbott, 2003, p. 650). Based on Abbott's comments, it appears that both a PCA and an EFA were conducted on the 1988 sample, and these analyses provided the foundation for the Abbott (2003) CFA that was conducted.

Abbott (2003) Confimatory Factor Analysis

Two CFA studies have been published on the POS since its initial development. Abbott (2003) conducted a series of CFAs using Amos 3.6 with

ML estimation (estimation methods are described in Chapter 2) and list-wise deletion of cases (ways of handing missing data, including listwise deletion, are discussed in Chapter 3) on the POS using a sample collected in 1998. The 1998 sample differed from the 1988 sample in several ways, but Abbott (2003) noted that "the differences tended to reflect general shifts within the social work profession" (p. 654). The initial CFA did not fit the data well. To improve the model fit, Abbott (2003) conducted additional analyses and made modifications to the model (like tailoring an article of clothing to get it to fit better). After several modifications, including dropping eight items and allowing for correlated errors for four pairs of items with similar content, an adequately fitting model was developed (Abbott, 2003).

Abbott (2003) concluded that the CFA "supported the construct validity[3] of the [four] value dimensions (factors) originally identified in the POS (Abbot, 1988). . . . Overall, the 1998 CFA provides additional evidence that reaffirms the construct of the 1988 generated factors" (p. 660). Interestingly, she also noted the question of whether positive and negative wording of items differentially impacted responses but that the issue was not a "major concern" (p. 663). Finally, she commented that additional work was still needed on the POS and that future studies should address a number of issues, including testing more diverse samples and examining and reporting reliability of the factors.

Because Abbott (2003) made a number of modifications to her model, what began as a CFA ended as an exploratory analysis, which in turn needs to be replicated. Even when model revisions are well-founded in the empirical literature and are theoretically based, once a model is re-specified (i.e., revised), it is no longer a confirmatory analysis and the resulting revised model needs to be confirmed in another sample (Brown, 2006). The second study of the POS was designed to confirm the CFA reported by Abbott (2003).

---

[3] Abbott's (2003) use of the term "construct validity" is in the broad sense of the term and, more specifically, could be referred to as structural (or factorial) validity using the terminology suggested by Koeske (1994).

Greeno, Hughes, Hayward, and Parker (2007) CFA

Greeno et al. (2007) conducted a series of CFAs on the POS using LISREL 8.7 with ML estimation and multiple imputation (multiple imputation is a way of addressing missing data that is discussed in Chapter 3). Data were collected in early 2006 using a mailed survey and a randomly selected sample of 234 NASW members (47.5% response rate). Although the 40-item version of the POS was used for the survey, the "initial CFA was conducted on the 32-item POS that resulted from Abbott's (2003) study. [The] first CFA model did not include the . . . error covariances from Abbott's 2003 study as the authors wanted to see if the error covariances were sample specific" (p. 487). This model did not fit well, and the authors removed four items with very low factor loadings; this resulted in a better fit, but there was still room for improvement. The final model reported included the 28 items and six error covariances suggested by the modification indices (i.e., data-driven suggestions about ways to improve the model fit); the six error covariances included the four identified in Abbott's (2003) model. The final model fit well, and Greeno and colleagues (2007) concluded that the "CFA supported a 28-item POS with six error correlations. The four subscales that Abbott (2003) proposed were also supported" (p. 488). However, the discriminant validity for the social responsibility and individual freedom factors is questionable given the high correlation (0.83) between these two factors.

Although Greeno et al.'s (2007) findings generally supported Abbott's (2003) findings, several modifications needed to be made to the model to achieve adequate fit, and consequently, a CFA of the Greeno et al. (2007) findings on an independent sample would strengthen their conclusions. As you may guess from this example, CFA may be thought of as a process —both within a single study as the model is modified to achieve adequate fit and across studies using the same measure as the latent structure of the measure is tested for fit across different samples or populations.

Chapter Summary

This chapter provides an introduction to the use of CFA in social work research and includes examples from the social work literature. CFA was also briefly compared to other data analysis techniques, including EFA, PCA, and SEM. Software for conducting CFA was briefly discussed and the software package used in this book was introduced. Finally, five published CFA articles were briefly discussed to provide examples of how CFA has been used in the social work literature.

Suggestions for Further Reading

Brown (2006) provides the first book-length treatment of CFA, which is a wonderful resource for more information on CFA, in general, and particularly some of the more technical aspects of CFA that are beyond the scope of the current book. Brown (2006) also provides more information on the five software packages mentioned in this chapter and CFA examples using each package. Kline (2005) and Raykov and Marcoulides (2006) provide good introductions to SEM; both provide a chapter on CFA and discuss other applications of SEM, including path analysis and latent change analysis. Kline (2005) also includes a useful chapter on "How to Fool Yourself with SEM." Byrne's (1998, 2001a, 2006) books on SEM with LISREL, Amos, and EQS (respectively) provide extensive information on using the software packages and multiple examples, several of which involve CFA. Byrne (2001b) compares Amos, EQS, and LISREL software for conducting CFAs.

There are many articles that provide overviews of SEM in specific content areas. For example, Hays, Revicki, and Coyne (2005) provide a brief overview and examples of SEM for health outcomes research, and Golob (2003) provides a similar overview and examples of SEM for travel behavior research. Given the number and variety of these articles now available, it is likely that readers can find a similar article in their area of interest.

Many multivariate statistics books (e.g., Stevens, 2002) provide introductions to PCA specifically, and others (e.g., Tabachnick & Fidell, 2007) provide a combined introduction to PCA and factor analysis, focusing on the similarities between the two analyses. Grimm and Yarnold (1994, 2000) provide nontechnical introductions to PCA, EFA, and CFA as well as SEM and testing the validity of measurement, respectively.

Koeske (1994) provides an excellent discussion of construct validity, including recommendations for the consistent use of validity terminology within social work research. Haynes, Richard, and Kubany (1995) discuss content validity as a component of construct validity; they also provide recommendations for examining and reporting evidence of content validity. See Shadish, Cook, and Campbell (2002) for an extensive discussion of validity as it relates to research design. Podsakoff et al. (2003) review the sources of common method biases, ways of addressing them, and information on correctly using CFA to control for method effects.

2

Creating a Confirmatory Factor Analysis Model

This chapter will focus on creating and specifying a confirmatory factor analysis (CFA) model, beginning with the role of theory and prior research in CFA. We will then discuss how a CFA model is specified, examining the role of observed and latent variables and model parameters, followed by a discussion of the importance of model identification, scaling latent variables, and estimation methods. We will end this chapter with a detailed example of testing a CFA model.

Specifying the Model

Theory and/or prior research are crucial to specifying a CFA model to be tested. As noted in Chapter 1, the one-factor solution of the Rosenberg Self-Esteem Scale was tested based on the conceptualization of self-esteem as a global (i.e., unitary) factor, although the existing exploratory factor analysis (EFA) work found two factors. Early in the process of measurement development, researchers may rely entirely on theory to develop a CFA model. However, as a measure is used over time, CFA can be used to replicate EFA or other analyses that have been conducted on the measure. In the Professional Opinion Scale (POS) example discussed in Chapter 1, Abbott's (2003) initial CFA was based both on underlying theory and an earlier EFA, whereas the Greeno et al. (2007) CFA was based on Abbott's (2003) earlier CFA work. Confirmatory factor analysis may not be an appropriate analysis to use if there is no strong underlying foundation on which to base the model, and more preliminary work, such as EFA or theory development, may be needed. This chapter includes many terms that are used in CFA, which will be defined here and in the Glossary. See Figure 2.1 for a basic CFA model with variables and parameters labeled.

Observed Variables

As discussed in Chapter 1, observed variables are those items that are directly observed, such as a response to a question. In CFA models, observed variables are represented by rectangles.

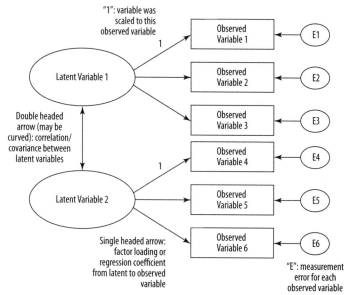

Figure 2.1 CFA Model With Parameters Labeled

Latent Variables

Latent variables are the underlying, unobserved constructs of interest. Ovals are used to represent latent variables in CFA models (sometimes circles are also used, but we will use ovals in this book). There are two types of latent variables: exogenous and endogenous. Exogenous variables are not caused by other variables in the model; they are similar to independent variables (IV), X, or predictors in regression analyses. Endogenous variables are–at least theoretically–caused by other variables, and in this sense they are similar to dependent variables (DV), Y, or outcome variables in regression analyses. In complex models, some variables may have both exogenous and endogenous functions.

CFA Model Parameters

Model parameters are the characteristics of the population that will be estimated and tested in the CFA. Relationships among observed and latent variables are indicated in CFA models by arrows going from the latent variables to the observed variables. The direction from the latent to the observed variable indicates the expectation that the underlying construct (e.g., depression) causes the observed variables (e.g., symptoms of unhappiness, feeling blue, changes in appetite, etc.). The factor loadings are the regression coefficients (i.e., slopes) for predicting the indicators from the latent factor. In general, the higher the factor loading the better, and typically loadings below 0.30 are not interpreted. As general rules of thumb, loadings above 0.71 are excellent, 0.63 very good, 0.55 good, 0.45 fair, and 0.32 poor (Tabachnick & Fidell, 2007). These rules of thumb are based on factor analyses, where factor loadings are correlations between the variable and factor, so squaring the loading yields a variance accounted for. Note that a loading of 0.71 squared would be 50% variance accounted for, whereas 0.32 squared would be 10% variance accounted for. In CFA, the interpretation of the factor loadings or regression coefficients is a little more complex if there is more than one latent variable in the model, but this basic interpretation will work for our purposes.

Whereas each indicator is believed to be caused by the latent factor, there may also be some unique variance in an indicator that is not accounted for by the latent factor(s). This unique variance is also known as measurement error, error variance, or indicator unreliability (see E1 to E6 in Figure 2.1).

Other parameters in a CFA model include factor variance, which is the variance for a factor in the sample data (in the unstandardized solution), and error covariances, which are correlated errors demonstrating that the indicators are related because of something other than the shared influence of the latent factor. Correlated errors could result from method effects (i.e., common measurement method such as self-report) or similar wording of items (e.g., positive or negative phrasing).

The relationship between two factors, or latent variables, in the model is a factor correlation in the completely standardized solution or a factor covariance in unstandardized solutions. Factor correlations represent the completely standardized solution in the same way that a Pearson's correlation is the "standardized" relationship between two variables (i.e., ranges from −1 to +1 and is unit-free—it does not include the original units of measurement). Similarly, factor covariances are unstandardized and include the original units of measurement just as variable covariances retain information about the original units of measurement and can range from negative infinity to positive infinity. Factor covariances or correlations are shown in CFA models as two-headed arrows (usually curved) between two latent variables.

Identification of the Model

Confirmatory factor analysis models must be identified to run the model and estimate the parameters. When a model is identified, it is possible to find unique estimates for each parameter with unknown values in the model, such as the factor loadings and correlations. For example, if we have an equation such as $a + b = 44$, there are an infinite number of combinations of values of a and b that could be used to solve this equation, such as $a = 3$ and $b = 41$ or $a = -8$ and $b = 52$. In this case, the model (or the equation) is underidentified because there are not enough known parameters to allow for a unique solution—in other words, there are more unknowns (*a* and *b*) than there are knowns (44) (Kline, 2005; Raykov & Marcoulides, 2006). Models must have degrees of freedom (*df*) greater than 0 (meaning we have more known than unknown parameters), and all latent variables must be scaled (which will be discussed later in this chapter) for models to be identified (Kline, 2005). When we meet these two conditions, the model can be solved and a unique set of parameters estimated. Models can be under-, just-, or overidentified.

Underidentified Models

Models are underidentified when the number of freely estimated parameters (i.e., unknowns) in the model is greater than the number of knowns. Underidentified models, such as the *a* + *b* = 44 example given earlier, cannot be solved because there are an infinite number of parameter estimates that will produce a perfect fit (Brown, 2006). In this situation we have negative *df*, indicating that the model cannot reach a unique solution because too many things are left to vary relative to the number of things that are known. The number of unknowns can be reduced by fixing some of the parameters to specific values. For example, if we set *b* = 4 in the aforementioned equation, then *a* can be solved because we know have more knowns (*b* and 44) than unknowns (*a*).

Just-Identified Models

Models are just-identified when the number of unknowns equals the number of knowns and *df* = 0. In this situation, there is one unique set of parameters that will perfectly fit and reproduce the data. Although this may initially sound like a great idea (What could be wrong with a perfectly fitting model?), in practice, perfectly fitting models are not very informative because they do not allow for model testing.

Overidentified Models

Models are overidentified when the number of unknowns is smaller than the number of knowns and *df* are greater than 0. Our *a* + *b* = 44 example stops working here because it is too simplistic to illustrate overidentified models, but Kline (2005) provides a nice example of how this works with sets of equations if you are interested in more information on identification of models. The difference between the number of knowns and unknowns is equal to the degrees of freedom (*df*) for the model. When a model is overidentified, goodness of fit can be evaluated and it is possible to test how well the model reproduces the input variance covariance matrix (Brown, 2006). Because we are interested in obtaining fit indices for CFA models, we want the models to be overidentified.

Scaling Latent Variables

As stated earlier, in addition to having *df* greater than 0, the second condition for model identification is that the latent variables have to be scaled. Scaling the latent variable creates one less unknown. Because latent variables are unobserved, they do not have a pre-defined unit of measurement; therefore, the researcher needs to set the unit of measurement. There are two ways to do this. One option is to make it the same as that of one of the indicator variables. The second option is to set the variance equal to 1 for the latent variable. In general, the first option is the more popular (Brown, 2006). Although these two options generally result in similar overall fit, they do not always do so and it is important to realize that the option chosen for scaling the latent variable may influence the standard errors and results of the CFA (Brown, 2006; Kline, 2005).

Scaling the latent variable (or setting its unit of measurement) is a little like converting currency. Imagine that you are creating a latent variable for cost of living across the United States, United Kingdom, and France, and you have three indicators—one in U.S. dollars, one in British pounds, and the other in Euros. Dollars, pounds, and Euros all have different scales of measurement, but the latent variable can be scaled (using the aforementioned option 1) to any one of these. If scaled to U.S. dollars, the latent variable will be interpretable in terms of dollars. But, the latent variable could also be scaled to either pounds or Euros—whichever will be most interpretable and meaningful for the intended audience.

Determining Whether a Model is Identified

As discussed earlier, you will want your CFA models to be overidentified so that you can test the fit of your model. Assuming that the latent variables have been properly scaled, the issue that will determine whether a model is identified is the number parameters to be estimated (i.e., the unknowns) relative to the number of known parameters. There are several rules of thumb available for testing the identification of models, such as the *t*-Rule and the Recursive Rule; however, these rules provide necessary but not sufficient guidance (Reilly, 1995), meaning that meeting the rule is necessary for identification, but the model may still be underidentified because of other issues. Fortunately for our purposes, SEM software used to conduct CFA will automatically test the identification of the model and will provide a message if the model is under- or just-identified, which should be sufficient for most situations.

Estimation Methods

"The objective of CFA is to obtain estimates for each parameter of the measurement model (i.e. factor loadings, factor variances and covariances, indicator error variances and possibly error covariances) that produce a predicted variance-covariance matrix (symbolized as Σ) that represents the sample variance-covariance matrix (symbolized as S) as closely as possible" (Brown, 2006, p. 72). In other words, in CFA we are testing whether the model fits the data. There are multiple estimation methods available for testing the fit of an overidentified model, and we briefly discuss several. The exact process of how the model is estimated using different estimation methods is beyond the scope of this book, but I will provide a general idea of how it works. Fitting a model is an iterative process that begins with an initial fit, tests how well the model fits, adjusts the model, tests the fit again, and so forth, until the model converges or fits well enough. This fitting process is done by the software used and will generally occur in a "black box" (i.e., it will not be visible to you).

This iterative fitting process is similar to having a garment, such as a wedding dress or suit, fitted. You begin with your best guess of what size should fit, and then the tailor assesses the fit and decides if adjustments are needed. If needed, the adjustments are made and then the garment is tried on again. This process continues until some fitting criteria are reached (i.e., the garment fits properly) or some external criteria (i.e., the wedding date) forces the process to stop. If the fitting criteria are reached, then the fit is said to converge and we have a well-fitting garment (or CFA model). But, if the fitting criteria are not reached, we may be forced to accept a poorly fitting garment (or CFA model) or to begin again with a new size or style (or a different CFA model). Just as there are multiple tailors available who will use slightly different fitting criteria, there are also multiple estimation methods available for CFA—each with its own advantages and disadvantages.

Some of the estimation methods that you may see in the literature include maximum likelihood (ML), weighted least squares (WLS), generalized least squares (GLS), and unweighted least squares (ULS). Although GLS and ULS are available in Amos 7.0 and may appear in the literature, both are used with multivariate normal data (Kline, 2005), and if data are multivariate normal, then ML is a better estimation procedure to use, so we will not discuss GLS and ULS. For this introductory text on CFA, we will limit our discussion to the best of the common estimation methods that are available in Amos 7.0.

Maximum Likelihood

Maximum likelihood (ML) is the most commonly used estimation method. Maximum likelihood "aims to find the parameter values that make the observed data most likely (or conversely maximize the likelihood of the parameters given the data)" (Brown, 2006, p. 73). Maximum likelihood estimation is similar (but not identical) to the ordinary least squares criterion used in multiple regression (Kline, 2005). It has several desirable statistical properties: *(1)* it provides standard errors (SEs) for each parameter estimate, which are used to calculate p-values (levels of significance), and confidence intervals, and *(2)* its fitting function is used to calculate many goodness-of-fit indices.

There are three key assumptions for ML estimation. First, this estimation procedure requires large sample sizes (sample size requirements will be discussed in more detail in Chapter 3). Second, indicators need to have continuous levels of measurement (i.e., no dichotomous, ordinal, or categorical indicator variables). Third, ML requires multivariate normally distributed indicators (procedures for assessing normality will be discussed in Chapter 3). ML estimation is robust to moderate violations, although extreme non-normality results in several problems: *(1)* underestimation of the SE, which inflates Type I error; *(2)* poorly behaved (inflated) χ^2 tests of overall model fit and underestimation of other fit indices (e.g., TLI and CFI, which will be discussed further in Chapter 4); and *(3)* incorrect parameter estimates. When there are severe violations of the assumptions, formulas are available for calculating robust SE estimates and the chi-square statistic as long as there are no missing data (see Gold, Bentler, & Kim, 2003). Importantly, the effects of non-normality worsen with smaller sample sizes (Brown, 2006). In addition, when the violations of the underlying assumptions are extreme, ML is prone to Heywood cases (i.e., parameter estimates with out-of-range values), such as negative error variances. In addition, minor misspecifications of the model may result in "markedly distorted solutions" (Brown, 2006, p. 75). Therefore, ML should not be used if the assumptions are violated.

Other Estimation Methods

If the model includes one or more categorical indicator variables or if there is extreme non-normality, ML is not appropriate to use and there are several alternative estimation methods available: *(1)* WLS, which is called asymptotically distribution-free (ADF) in Amos 7.0; *(2)* robust weighted least squares (WLSMV); and *(3)* ULS (Brown, 2006). However, each of these estimation methods has limitations, as discussed below. For non-normal continuous indicators, ML with robust SE and χ^2 (MLM) can be used. At this time, the Mplus program has the best options for handling categorical data because of the availability of the WLSMV estimator (Brown, 2006).

Of the estimation methods that are broadly available, including in Amos, ADF "estimates the degree of both skew and kurtosis in the raw data" and therefore makes no assumptions about the distribution of the data (Kline, 2005, p. 196). Although this addresses the problem of non-normality in the data, a drawback of this approach is that it generally requires very large sample sizes of 200 to 500 for simple models and thousands of cases for complex models (Kline, 2005, p. 196). In addition to the sample size requirements, Brown (2006) notes that ADF or WLS does not perform well with categorical data, especially when samples are not sufficiently large.

Gold et al. (2003) compared ML and ADF estimation methods for non-normal incomplete data and found that direct ML (the form of ML that can handle missing data, which is available in Amos and other software packages) performs better than ADF with pairwise deletion, regardless of missing data mechanism (p. 73). Gold et al. (2003) concluded that ADF should not be used with missing data, and if there are missing data, even when there is non-normality, "ML methods are still preferable, although they should be used with robust standard errors and rescaled chi-square statistics" (p. 74). Savalei and Bentler (2005) also concluded that direct ML is generally recommended when there are missing data and non-normality. Missing data and normality will be discussed further in Chapter 3.

In Amos Graphics 7.0, the available estimation methods are ML, GLS, ULS, scale-free least squares, and ADF. Only ML can be used if there are missing data. If there are missing data and one of the other estimation methods is needed, then some form of data imputation needs to be done before the other estimation method can be used in Amos. Readers who are likely to have problematic data may want to consider using a software package other than Amos.

Testing a Confirmatory Factor Analysis Model Example

In this section, we will use Amos 7.0 to test a CFA model using the Maslach Burnout Inventory (MBI; Maslach, Jackson, & Leiter, 1996). Brief instructions for using Amos 7.0 to conduct this analysis are provided in Appendix A. The data for this example are from a study of U.S. Air Force Family Advocacy Program (FAP) workers (Bean, Harrington, & Pintello, 1998; Harrington, Bean, Pintello, & Mathews, 2001). The sample includes 139 FAP workers and the response rate for the survey was 74%. Before continuing, it is important to note that this sample size is considered medium (Kline, 2005) for this analysis (although one can find published CFA articles with similar and even smaller size samples). Therefore, it is offered only as an example data set that readers can play with, not one from which conclusions should be drawn. Ideally, the sample size would be larger, as will be discussed in Chapter 3.

Specifying the Model

The MBI was developed in the late 1970s by Maslach and Jackson to measure burnout in human service workers. It is considered the most widely accepted and often used self-report index of burnout in research studies and employee assessment. This 22-item self-report scale treats burnout as a continuous variable that can be divided into three components: emotional exhaustion (EE), depersonalization (DP), and personal accomplishment (PA). Each item is measured on a seven-point Likert-type scale assessing the frequency of occurrence (ranging from 0 = never to 6 = a few times a day). For EE and DP, higher scores indicate higher levels of burnout, with higher levels of emotional exhaustion and depersonalization, respectively. For PA, higher scores indicate lower levels of burnout and higher levels of personal accomplishment. Maslach suggests that each subscale be scored separately rather than as a composite because this provides the best representation of the multidimensional nature of burnout as a construct (Schaufeli & Van Dierendonck, 1995).

As discussed earlier, specifying the model to be tested should be based on theory and prior research. There has been extensive work on the MBI, including a CFA on the three-factor MBI in a sample of child welfare workers (Drake & Yadama, 1995). There has also been extensive debate about how the three factors are related to burnout, whether they are all components of burnout, or whether EE is really the indicator of burnout, with PA and DP being related but separate constructs.

Like Drake and Yadama (1995), we will begin by testing the three-factor structure of the MBI as defined by Maslach et al. (1996). The observed variables for the model are the 22 items that participants responded to, and the latent variables are the three factors identified by Maslach et al. (1996). The indicators for each latent variable were chosen based on scoring instructions provided by Maslach and colleagues (1996). Because the three factors are believed to be related to each other, covariances (or correlations) among the latent variables are included in the model (shown as the two headed curved arrows in Figure 2.2 below).

Identification of the Model

The MBI CFA model is overidentified with 206 *df*, which means that there are fewer parameters to be estimated than there are known parameters. Each latent variable is scaled, with the path coefficient for one observed variable being set to "1" for each latent variable.

Estimation Method

Maximum likelihood (ML) estimation was used for this model. The MBI observed variables can be treated as continuous and the data are approximately normally distributed (data considerations will be discussed in Chapter 3), making ML a reasonable estimation method to use. It should be noted that the sample size for this example is smaller ($n = 139$) than desired for this or any other CFA estimation procedure, but these data are used for example purposes only.

Model Fit

All the observed variables are significantly related to the latent variables and EE and DP are significantly correlated as expected. However, contrary to

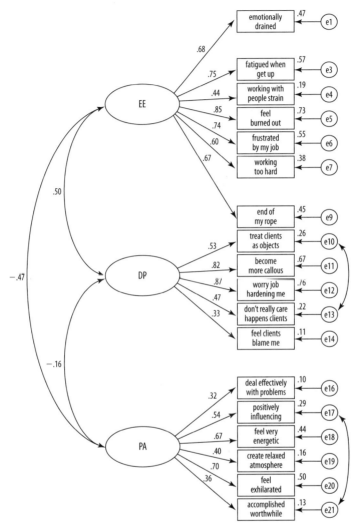

Figure 2.2 Respecified MBI CFA Model Standardized Output (Amos 7.0 Graphics)

expectations, PA and DP are not correlated ($r = -0.127$; $p = 0.261$), and PA and EE are not correlated ($r = -0.226$; $p = 0.056$). Although the model tested was based on a well-developed and tested measure, the model does not fit as well as desired. We will discuss assessing model fit in detail in Chapter 4.

Model Respecification

Drake and Yadama (1995) also found that the 22-item, three-factor MBI CFA did not fit well. To respecify their model (respecification will be discussed in more detail in Chapter 4, but briefly to respecify means to revise), they examined intercorrelations among items and deleted two items (2 and 16) that were very similar in content and highly correlated with other items. Drake and Yadama (1995) also examined squared multiple correlations and dropped two items (4 and 21) with very low squared multiple correlations. Finally, modification indices suggested that allowing the error terms to be correlated for items 5 and 15 on the DP scale and items 9 and 19 on the PA scale would improve model fit; because both of these changes seemed reasonable, the error terms were allowed to covary. Drake and Yadama's final model fit well and indicators loaded on latent variables as expected.

Using Drake and Yadama's (1996) prior work as guidance, the MBI CFA was respecified according to their final model (i.e., 18 items, three factors, and adding two error covariances). Similarly to Drake and Yadama's (1996) findings, the respecified model fits much better than the original 22-item, three-factor model. Figure 2.2 shows the standardized output for the final model. All regression weights in the model are significant and indicators load on the expected latent variables, EE and DP are significantly correlated ($p < 0.0005$), and EE and PA are significantly correlated ($p = 0.013$); the correlation between PA and DP is nonsignificant ($p = 0.193$).

Conclusion

The respecified model fit the data adequately, supporting the modified structure reported by Drake and Yadama (1995). The changes made to the model by Drake and Yadama (1995) were data-driven, and they noted that their findings should be considered preliminary with further CFA work needed with other samples. The findings in this example cautiously (because of the small sample size) suggest support for the 18-item model Drake and Yadama (1995) reported, rather than the original Maslach et al. (1996) 22-item model.

Chapter Summary

This chapter focused on creating and specifying a CFA model, including the use of theory and prior research. Observed and latent variables, CFA model parameters, model identification, and scaling the latent variables were defined, and conventions for drawing CFA models were presented. Estimation methods used in the CFA literature were briefly discussed, and ML estimation was discussed in detail. Finally, a detailed example of a CFA on the MBI was presented.

Suggestions for Further Reading

See Arbuckle (2006) for much more information on using Amos 7.0 Graphics. Byrne's (1998, 2001a, 2006) books on structural equation modeling with LISREL, Amos, and EQS (respectively) provide a number of CFA examples using these software packages. Reilly (1995) provides instructions and examples using the Rank Rule to determine whether a CFA model will be identified. Brown (2006) provides more information on how the estimation methods and fitting functions work. See Drake and Yadama (1995) for more detail on how they conducted the CFA that was replicated in this chapter. See Gold, Bentler, and Kim (2003) and Savalei and Bentler (2005) for more information on the Monte Carlo studies they conducted to compare ML and ADF estimation methods with missing data and non-normality.

3

Requirements for Conducting Confirmatory Factor Analysis
Data Considerations

This chapter will focus on the requirements for conducting a confirmatory factor analysis (CFA), including reviewing issues around missing data, normality, categorical variables, and sample size adequacy. Because these issues are quite technical, a brief introduction and suggestions for ways to address each issue, as well as suggested readings for additional information, will be provided.

Missing Data

Most data sets have some missing data, but researchers often fail to indicate the amount of missing data and how missing data were handled in the analyses. Missing data can affect any kind of data analysis, including confirmatory factor analysis (CFA). Missing data can result in reduced power if cases with missing values are dropped from an analysis; for studies that plan for the necessary sample size using an a priori power analysis, missing data can result in an underpowered study and nonsignificant findings. If there is a pattern to the missing data, then there may be misleading results and the possibility of erroneous implications being drawn from the findings. There are several common ways of handling missing data, and each has implications for analyses—using different methods of addressing missing data can result in different findings, therefore it is extremely important to report how missing data were handled. In addition, it is important to note that the amount of missing data may be less important than the pattern of missingness (Savalei & Bentler, 2005; Tabachnick & Fidell, 2007).

The best way to handle missing data depends on the type of missing data that exists in the study. There are three types of missing data: *(1)* missing completely at random, *(2)* missing at random, and *(3)* nonignorable or missing not at random. Data can be *missing completely at random* (MCAR), in which case the probability of missing data is unrelated to values of Y and other variables in the data set (Brown, 2006). Researchers can test whether data are MCAR (Brown, 2006). Data are *missing at random* (MAR) when the probability of missing data on Y may depend on X but is not related to the value of Y when X is held constant. In other words, MAR data may be predictable from other variables in the data set. For example, in a long survey of adults over the age of 65 years, a researcher may find that age is related to not answering all the questions at the end of the survey, and it could just be that the oldest participants were more likely to become fatigued and stop answering the questions. MAR is more likely to hold in applied research than MCAR, but it is impossible to test for in applied data (Brown, 2006). Fortunately, mistakenly assuming that data are MAR often has only a small impact on standard errors and estimates (Schafer & Graham, 2002). *Nonignorable* missing data occur when data are missing in a predictable pattern that is related to other variables. For example, if respondents who do not report their income have higher incomes than those who do report their income, then missing data on income are nonignorable.

It is important to know how your software handles missing data. Several data analysis software packages, including SPSS and SAS, generally default to dropping all cases with any missing data on variables included in an analysis (this process is known as listwise deletion). This default process can result in the loss of a large number of cases without the researcher's awareness. Amos 7.0 will automatically address missing data when using maximum likelihood estimation, and whereas this may sound ideal, it can be problematic if there is a great deal of missing data or if it is nonignorable. No matter how your software addresses missing data, it is necessary to check for the extent and pattern of missing data before conducting confirmatory factor analysis (CFA) or any other analysis. It is also important for the researcher to decide how to handle missing data, but unfortunately, none of the options are ideal, and sometimes the researcher is forced to choose between several bad options (Tabachnick & Fidell, 2007). We discuss some of the available options for addressing missing data below.

Checking for Missing Data

You can check for missing data using frequencies and descriptive statistics in any data analysis software package, and the SPSS Missing Values Analysis (MVA), in particular, is designed to identify patterns of missing data and has several options for imputing (i.e., replacing) missing values (Tabachnick & Fidell, 2007). MVA will provide extensive information on both the amount and pattern of missing data. As mentioned in Chapter 2 when discussing estimation methods, it appears that the pattern of missing data is more important than the amount of missing data. There are no guidelines for how much missing data is too much. Tabachnick and Fidell (2007) suggest that for large data sets with 5% or less of the data points missing at random, then the problems are unlikely to be serious and any method for handling missing data should be ok.

Deletion of Cases With Missing Data

Two of the most common ways of handling missing data in general are listwise and pairwise deletion of cases. With listwise deletion, only cases with complete data are retained and used in data analyses. Listwise deletion is very common and is often the default option in software packages (e.g., SPSS and SAS). Pairwise deletion retains more data than listwise deletion because cases are only dropped from correlations in which they did not answer one or both of the variables, rather than being dropped from all correlations because one response was missing. Pairwise deletion includes cases for correlations (or covariances) for all pairs of variables with valid responses.

Listwise deletion results in the same sample size for all correlations or covariances produced for a matrix, whereas pairwise deletion generally results in different sample sizes for different correlations or covariances, depending on the pattern of missing data. In general, deletion of cases with missing data is not recommended. Both listwise and pairwise deletion can result in a loss of power. Additionally, when the data are not MCAR, case deletion procedures may result in biased parameter estimates, standard errors, and test statistics. For minor departures from MCAR, the bias may be minor, but the extent of the bias is hard to determine (Schafer & Graham, 2002). Finally, even when the missing data are MCAR, estimates produced with listwise or pairwise deletion are less efficient than when other methods of handling missing data are used (Enders, 2001).

Mean Substitution

One approach to handling missing data is to substitute the variable mean for all missing values on that variable. This used to be a very common approach, and it is still an option for handling missing data in many procedures, such as factor analysis, in SPSS and other software packages. However, this is not a good approach, and it should be avoided (Shafer & Graham, 2002).

Imputation of Missing Data

Another method for handling missing data is to impute missing values before the data are used for the CFA analysis. There are several ways to do this, but one of the more common is the expectation maximization (EM) algorithm available in SPSS. Expectation maximization employs a two-step iterative process. In the estimation step, missing values are replaced with predicted values based on a series of regression equations. In the

M step, maximum likelihood (ML) estimates are calculated as if the data were complete (Enders, 2001). These two steps are repeated (this is the iterative part of the process) until the solution converges, meaning that the covariance matrices produced at subsequent steps are extremely similar. At the end of this process, missing data can be estimated (i.e., imputed), resulting in what looks like a complete data set. However, note that the imputation does not include a random error component that would be present if the data were complete. Therefore, standard errors generated from the imputed dataset may be somewhat negatively biased, and correct estimates must be calculated using bootstrap techniques (Enders, 2001). However, as noted below under Estimation Methods for Non-Normal Data, bootstrapping is not recommended; therefore, whereas SPSS MVA is useful for examining missing data patterns, the EM procedure is not universally recommended for imputing missing data.

Recommended Strategies for Handling Missing Data

Although listwise and pairwise deletion are commonly used to handle missing data, they are not recommended. Two strategies that are recommended for handling missing data when conducting a CFA are maximum likelihood (which is called several different things, including direct ML, full information ML, or ML estimation based on all available data) and Bayesian multiple imputation (Allison, 2003; Brown, 2006; Schafer & Graham, 2002). Both approaches use all available data and produce parameter estimates, standard errors (SEs), and test statistics that are consistent (i.e., unbiased) and efficient (i.e., less data are lost) when MCAR or MAR holds and data have a multivariate normal distribution (Brown, 2006). Savalei and Bentler's (2005) findings suggest direct ML also works well with some non-normality. Amos 7.0 computes direct ML estimates by default whether there are missing or complete data. However, it is important to note that Amos assumes the data are missing at random and should not be used if the missingness is not random (Arbuckle, 2006b). In addition, direct ML should only be used when the assumptions for ML have been met; this method is not appropriate if the data are extremely non-normally distributed (Enders, 2001). The direct ML approach uses all available information, but not all fit indices (e.g., goodness-of-fit index [GFI]) can be computed with this approach and it may produce indefinite covariance matrices. When using direct ML, missing values are not imputed, but parameters are estimated as if complete data were available (Enders, 2001).

If the assumptions for ML have not been met and another fitting function is needed, then multiple imputation is recommended (Allison, 2003; Brown, 2006). Multiple imputation involves multiple steps and is beyond the scope of this book. Allison (2003) cautions that multiple imputation can be used in most situations, but the results vary every time you use it and there are multiple ways to implement multiple imputation, which can be challenging for novices. If the missing data are non-ignorable, then there are extensions of both ML and multiple imputation that can be used, but they are difficult to implement, vulnerable to misspecification, and should only be used when the researcher understands the missing data mechanism. However, it is important to note that even when the data are not missing at random, methods that assume the data are missing at random, such as direct ML, can produce good results (Allison, 2003).

Normality

Multivariate normality is assumed for most CFA estimation methods, including maximum likelihood (as discussed Chapter 2). Multivariate normality means all variables are univariate normally distributed, the distribution of any pair of variables is bivariate normal, and all pairs of variables have linear and homoscedastic scatterplots (Kline, 2005). Although it is difficult to assess all aspects of multivariate normality, checking for univariate normality and outliers will detect most cases of multivariate non-normality (Kline, 2005).

Univariate Normality

A non-normal distribution may be detected because of significant skew or kurtosis. Skew is a measure of how asymmetric a unimodal distribution is. If most of the scores are below the mean, then the distribution is positively skewed, whereas if most of the scores are above the mean, then the distribution is negatively skewed. Kurtosis is a measure of how well the shape of the bell conforms to that of a normal distribution. Positive kurtosis, or a leptokurtic distribution, occurs when the middle of the distribution has a higher peak than expected for a normal distribution (imagine someone trapped under a normal distribution who is leaping up and down trying to get out—they would bump up the middle of the distribution). Negative kurtosis, or a platykurtic distribution, occurs when the middle of the distribution is flatter than expected for a normal distribution (imagine a platypus with a slightly rounded but flattish back).

You can test whether a variable has significant skew or kurtosis by dividing the unstandardized skewness or kurtosis index by its corresponding standard error; this ratio is interpreted as a z-test of skew or kurtosis (Kline, 2005). Therefore, ratios greater than 1.96 would have p-value less than 0.05, and ratios greater than 2.58 would have p-value less than 0.01, indicating significant skewness or kurtosis in the data. However, in large samples, these tests may be overly sensitive to non-normality. An alternative to the ratio test is to interpret the absolute values of the skew and kurtosis indexes, with absolute values of skew greater than 3.0 indicating the distribution is extremely skewed and absolute values of kurtosis greater than 10.0 suggesting a problem; values greater than 20.0 indicate a potentially serious problem with kurtosis (Kline, 2005).

Outliers

Outliers are extreme or very unusual cases that can bias estimators and significance tests (Yuan & Bentler, 2001). Cases can be univariate or multivariate outliers. Univariate outliers have extreme scores on one variable and can be detected by examining z-scores; cases with z-scores greater than 3.0 in absolute value are unusual and may be outliers (Kline, 2005). However, in very large data sets, using z-scores greater than 3.0 may be too conservative, and using a cut-point of 4.0 or greater in absolute value may more accurately identify outliers.

Multivariate outliers may have extreme scores on more than one variable or may have an unusual combination of values, but none of the individual variables have extreme scores. For example, in a survey of job satisfaction and burnout among social workers, you might ask for respondents' age and work experience measured in number of years in the same job. If the age range for the sample is from 23 to 70 years, and the number of years in the same job ranges from 1 to 35, a 58-year-old with 35 years experience in the same job may not be an outlier on either age or job experience, but the combination of being 58 years old with 35 years of experience in the same job may be unusual enough that the respondent is a multivariate outlier. Mahalanobis distance (D) can be used to identify multivariate outliers; roughly speaking, D indicates how unusual a case is on the set of variables compared with the sample centroids (i.e., means or mid-points) for all the variables. Significance tests for D can be obtained from several software packages, including SPSS, and a conservative significance level ($p < 0.001$) is recommended for this test (Kline, 2005).

Outliers can be problematic because they may cause non-normality and may result in Heywood cases (Brown, 2006). Problematic outliers can be dropped from the analyses (Meyers, Gamst, & Guarino, 2006) if the sample size is sufficiently large to allow that as an option; however, if outliers are dropped, then you should consider how this affects the generalizability of your findings. Another option is to winsorize the outliers (Shete et al., 2004)—that is, recode the variable for the extreme case so that the case still has the highest score but no longer one that is so extreme. For example, in a sample with incomes ranging from $27,000 to $123,000 for all cases but one, which has an income of $376,000, you might recode the case with the highest income from $376,000 to $125,000—a value that is still the highest in the data set, but not one that is so extreme as to distort all other statistics. Winsorization can reduce skewness and platykurtosis (Shete et al., 2004).

Data Checking with SPSS and Amos

Univariate normality is easy to assess in any data analysis software package. Because this book is intended as an initial introduction to CFA, it is assumed that readers may be more familiar with general data analysis software (such as SAS or SPSS) than with SEM software (such as Amos). Therefore, the easiest way to examine univariate normality may be through descriptive statistics in whichever data analysis software program you are most comfortable using. For the JSS dataset (which will be discussed in detail in Chapter 4), the descriptive statistics shown in Table 4.1 in Chapter 4 were generated in SPSS. Amos 7.0 does not provide tests of univariate and multivariate normality for data sets with missing data; however, normality checks are available for complete data (such as those shown in Table 4.3 in Chapter 4).[1]

Estimation Methods for Non-Normal Data

Although ML estimation assumes that the data are multivariate normal and is robust to minor non-normality, it is particularly sensitive to excessive kurtosis (Brown, 2006). Using the rules of thumb provided by Kline (2005), this suggests that absolute values of kurtosis indices greater than 20.0 may be problematic with ML estimation. If extreme non-normality exists, it is better not to use ML. The best approach for handling extreme non-normality is to use the robust ML (MLM) estimator (Brown, 2006), but this estimator is not available in Amos 7.0. If you are using Amos 7.0, the best option is direct ML with robust estimators (see Yuan, Bentler & Zhang, 2005). Other approaches to non-normality, such as bootstrapping, item parceling, and data transformation are not recommended (Brown, 2006) and therefore are not discussed here.

Levels of Measurement

Data can be categorical, ordinal, or continuous. Most of the estimation methods used for CFA assume continuous data, but it is not always clear whether the types of response options used for many measures can be

---

[1] For more information on obtaining the normality statistics in Amos, see the "NormalityCheck Method" under Amos Help.

treated as continuous. Some variables are clearly categorical (such as race or ethnicity), and others are clearly continuous (such as age in years or income in dollars). However, many instruments use Likert-type response options, where respondents are asked to rate how much they agree or disagree with a statement on a multiple-point scale. When there are only a few response options (e.g., very, somewhat, or not satisfied), treating the variables as continuous—that is, ignoring their categorical or ordinal nature—can result in biased results with some estimation methods, such as ML (Raykov & Marcoulides, 2006). However, it may be possible to treat the variables as continuous when there are at least five response categories, the sample size is sufficiently large, and the data are approximately normally distributed (i.e., no extreme skewness or kurtosis) (Cohen, Cohen, West, & Aiken, 2003). (The JSS dataset, which will be discussed in Chapter 4, includes Likert-type variables that meet these criteria and are treated as continuous variables.) ML assumes continuous data are being used; therefore, another estimator must be used for categorical variables. Asymptotically distribution-free (ADF) estimation can be used with categorical data in very large samples, but MLM (i.e., direct ML) is preferred (Brown, 2006).

Sample Size Requirements

Although researchers agree that the larger the sample size, the better for CFA, there is no universal agreement about how large is large enough. In addition, some estimation procedures (such as ADF used for non-normal data) require even larger sample sizes than are necessary with normally distributed data and ML estimation (Lee & Song, 2004). Unfortunately, there is no easy way to determine the sample size needed for CFA. The four existing approaches are briefly discussed: rules of thumb, the Satorra–Saris method, the MacCallum approach, and Monte Carlo studies.

Rules of Thumb

There are some very rough guidelines for sample sizes: less than 100 is considered "small" and may only be appropriate for very simple models; 100 to 200 is "medium" and may be an acceptable minimum sample size if the model is not too complex; and greater than 200 is "large", which is probably acceptable for most models (Kline, 2005). Small sample sizes may result in technical problems when running the analysis (such as non-convergence or improper solutions) and low power (Kline, 2005).

For CFA models with small or medium sample sizes, Kline (2005, citing Marsh & Hau, 1999) suggests using indicators with good psychometric properties and standardized factor loadings greater than 0.60, imposing equality constraints (i.e., forcing parameters to be equal rather than freely estimated) on the unstandardized loadings of indicators on the same factor, and using parcels (i.e., groups of indicators) for categorical items. However, as noted earlier, Brown (2006) recommends against using item parcels or any of the multiple rules of thumb for determining what the sample size should be.

Lee and Song (2004) conducted a simulation study comparing ML and Bayesian estimation with small sample sizes. They concluded that ML is not recommended with small sample sizes, even when data are normally distributed; however, the Bayesian approach is recommended with small sample sizes as long as the sample size is two to three times as large as the number of unknown parameters to be estimated. Performance of the Bayesian approach improves with larger samples and "produces accurate parameter estimates and reliable goodness-of-fit test" (Lee & Song, 2004, p. 680) when the ratio of sample size to parameters is 4:1 or 5:1. Lee and Song's (2004) findings suggest that under some cases, these rough rules of thumb may provide reasonable guidance for sample size estimates, at least for normally distributed data. However, Muthén and Muthén (2002) caution that no rule of thumb is applicable across all situations because the "sample size needed for a study depends on many factors, including the size of the model, distribution of the variables, amount of missing data, reliability of the variables, and strength of the relations among the variables" (pp. 599–600). Finally, Gignac (2006) suggests that sample size requirements should be treated as recommendations to be tested and that in some cases SEM may be appropriate in sample sizes as small as 100.

Satorra–Saris Method

The Satorra–Saris (1985; Saris & Satorra, 1993) method is a model-based quantitative approach, which is better than the rules of thumb, but has several disadvantages, so it is not recommended (Brown, 2006). The Satorra–Saris method is only mentioned here because readers may see it referenced in the literature.

MacCallum Approach

MacCallum and Hong (1997) extended the work of MacCallum, Brown, and Sugawara (1996) and concluded that power analysis should be based on the root mean square error of estimation fit index, rather than the GFI (these are goodness of fit indices that will be discussed in Chapter 4) because of "the undesirable influence of degrees of freedom on GFI-based [power] analyses" (p. 209). MacCallum, Widaman, Preacher, and Hong (2001) examined the role of model error in sample size requirements for factor analysis and concluded that the traditional sample size rules of thumb are of limited value and EFA can work well when communalities are high—almost regardless of sample size, model error, or level of over-determination of the factors (p. 636).

Preacher and MacCallum (2002) extend this conclusion and state that "As long as communalities are high, the number of expected factors is relatively small, and model error is low (a condition which often goes hand-in-hand with high communalities), researchers and reviewers should not be overly concerned about small sample sizes" (p. 160). However, if communalities are low and factors are not highly overdetermined, then much larger sample sizes are needed. Overall, they found that no general recommendations about sample size could be made. Although these studies involved EFA, the authors concluded that the results should be equally valid for CFA as long as the CFA is "not badly misspecified" (MacCallum et al., 2001, p. 636).

Monte Carlo Approach

Muthén and Muthén (2002) demonstrated the use of a Monte Carlo study with Mplus to identify the appropriate sample size and to determine power for CFA. Monte Carlo studies are conducted by generating data from a population with hypothesized parameter values. Multiple samples are drawn, the model is estimated for each sample, and the "parameter values and standard errors are averaged over the samples" (p. 600). Before conducting the Monte Carlo study, the researcher must decide on the model to be tested and select population values for every parameter in the model. Estimates may come from theory or prior research, with the best estimates coming from prior studies. Then the researcher must decide how many samples will be drawn (i.e., how many replications there will be) and select multiple seed values (i.e., the starting points for the random selection of the samples). There must be enough replications to achieve stable results, and Muthén and Muthén (2002) used 10,000 replications in their study. Before you panic and decide that this is overwhelming and impossible, remember that the computer software is going to do the vast majority of the work for you! You will not actually be running 10,000 replications—you will be programming the software to do it for you. Muthén and Muthén (2002) provide the Mplus files for conducting the analyses they report.

A major advantage of the Monte Carlo approach is that it allows the researcher to consider important aspects of the data, such as missingness and normality. Patterns and amounts of missing data and skewness and kurtosis can be specified. In their Monte Carlo study, Muthén and Muthén (2002) used ML estimation; an estimator that is robust to nonnormality was used with the non-normal data to estimate the SEs. For their CFA model, Muthén and Muthén (2002) found a sample size of 150 was needed when the data were normally distributed and there were no missing data. The necessary sample size increased to 175 when there were randomly missing data, 265 for non-normal complete data, and 315 when the data were non-normal and had some missingness. These findings clearly indicate the impact of the distribution and missingness of the data on sample size requirements needed for adequate power.

Chapter Summary

This chapter focused on data considerations and assumptions for conducting CFA. Types of missing data and checking for and addressing missing data were addressed. Normality was also discussed, including how to assess univariate and multivariate normality as well as estimation methods for non-normal data. Levels of measurement and associated estimation methods were briefly mentioned. Finally, approaches to determining the sample size required for CFA, such as rules of thumb, the Satorra–Saris method, the MacCallum approach, and the Monte Carlo approach were introduced.

Suggestions for Further Reading

Allison (2003) discusses techniques for handling missing data for SEM and provides a detailed discussion of multiple imputation. Brown (2006) provides more information on how to test whether data are missing at random and on how to conduct multiple imputation to address missing data. Enders (2001) reviews three maximum likelihood algorithms for handling missing data: multiple-group approach, direct ML, and EM. Graham (2003) discusses the advantages of including "auxiliary" variables "that are correlated with variables containing missingness" (p. 80), which can improve estimation of structural equation models; he also provides examples and syntax for doing this using Amos. Schafer and Graham (2002) review the methods available for handling missing data and describe the strengths and limitations of each method; several of the methods they review are not recommended or are not typically applicable for CFA (e.g., ipsative mean imputation), so they are not discussed in this book, but readers may find those methods useful for other types of data analyses. The details of running a Monte Carlo study to determine sample size and power are beyond the scope of this introductory text, but interested readers can see Brown (2006, pp. 420–429) for an introduction to this approach and Muthén and Muthén (2002) for how to use M*plus* to conduct a Monte Carlo study.

4

Assessing Confirmatory
Factor Analysis Model Fit
and Model Revision

This chapter will focus on how to determine whether a model fits well, including a discussion of the various fit indices available, which ones to use, and thresholds for determining acceptable fit. We will also examine how to revise a model that does not fit well, including incorporating theory-based changes and the use of modification indices. Finally, a detailed confirmatory factor analysis (CFA) example is presented that includes a discussion of all the aspects of specifying, testing, assessing, and revising the model.

Assessment of Model Fit

There are several different goodness-of-fit indices, and most of them can be best viewed as describing the lack of fit of the model to the data. Each type of fit index provides different information about model fit (or non-fit), so researchers generally report multiple fit indices when evaluating model fit. Although there are many recommendations for which fit indices to report and their corresponding criteria for what indicates adequate or good fit (e.g., Kline, 2005; Raykov, Tomer, & Nesselroade, 1991), we will use Brown's (2006) recommendations because they are based on both popularity of use in the research literature and performance in Monte Carlo research. Brown identifies three categories of fit indices: *(1)* absolute fit indices, *(2)* parsimony correction indices, and *(3)* comparative fit indices. In addition to these three categories of fit indices, we will also briefly discuss predictive fit indices.

Absolute Fit Indices

Absolute fit indices test the hypothesis that $\Sigma = S$—that is, whether the predicted variance-covariance matrix (Σ) is equal to the sample variance–covariance matrix (S). In other words, absolute fit indices answer the question "Is the residual (unexplained) variance appreciable?" (Chau et al., 2006, p. 1012). The most common absolute fit index is the model chi-square (χ^2), which tests whether the model fits exactly in the population. There are multiple limitations to the model chi-square (e.g., it is dependent on sample size and will almost always be significant with large samples), but it is useful for testing nested models, which are discussed later in this chapter. Other absolute fit indices include the Root Mean Square Residual (RMR), which is the average discrepancy between the covariances in the input matrix and the covariances predicted by the model. Because the RMR is affected by the metric of the input variables, it can be difficult to interpret. The Standardized Root Mean Square Residual (SRMR) is based on the discrepancy between the correlations in the input matrix and the correlations predicted by the model, which is standardized and therefore easier to interpret and, consequently, is generally preferred over the RMR (Brown, 2006).

Parsimony Correction Indices

The parsimony correction indices incorporate a penalty for poor parsimony, therefore more complex models will be viewed as having poorer fit. The root mean square error of approximation (RMSEA) tests the extent to which the model fits *reasonably* well in the population; it is sensitive to model complexity, but unlike the model chi-square, it is relatively insensitive to sample size. Close fit (CFit) indicates the probability (p) that RMSEA is less than or equal to 0.05 (Brown, 2006).

Comparative Fit Indices

Comparative fit indices are used to evaluate the fit of a model relative to a more restricted, nested baseline model. Examples include the comparative fit index (CFI) and the Tucker-Lewis index (TLI) or non-normed fit index (NNFI).

Predictive Fit Indices

Predictive fit indices "assess model fit in *hypothetical* replication samples of the same size and randomly drawn from the same population as the researcher's original sample … these indexes may be seen as population based rather than sample based" (Kline, 2005, p. 142). The Akaike information criterion (AIC) is used with maximum likelihood (ML) estimation and "favors simpler models" so, in some senses, it is also a parsimony fit index (Kline, 2005, p. 142). The AIC is generally used to compare between two (or more) non-nested models tested on the same data set. A smaller AIC suggests that the model is more likely to replicate, has fewer parameters, and fits better; therefore, when comparing models, the one with the smaller AIC is chosen as the "better" model. The expected cross-validation index (ECVI) is also used when comparing models and will result in the same rank ordering of models as the AIC (Kline, 2005). Similarly to the AIC, the ECVI is population-based and parsimony adjusted. The predictive fit indices are used for comparing models, so unlike the other categories of fit indices, there are no guidelines for what represents acceptable fit.

Recommendations for Assessing Acceptable Model Fit

There are multiple guidelines available for "acceptable" model fit. Brown (2006) recommends RMSEA close to 0.06 or less; SRMR close to 0.08

or less; CFI close to 0.95 or greater; and TLI close to 0.95 or greater. It is important to note that these are not rigid guidelines, and Brown comments that his use of "close to" is purposeful. Kline (2005) recommends that model chi-square, RMSEA, 90% confidence interval for RMSEA, CFI, and SRMR be reported. According to Kline (2005) "RMSEA $\leq$ .05 indicates close approximate fit, values between .05 and .08 suggest reasonable error of approximation, and RMSEA $\geq$ .10 suggests poor fit" (p. 139). CFI "greater than roughly .90 may indicate reasonably good fit of the researcher's model" (Kline, 2005, p. 140), and SRMR values "less than .10 are generally considered favorable" (Kline, 2005, p. 141). It is important to note that although Brown (2006) and Kline (2005) recommend reporting several of the same fit indices, their criteria for acceptable fit are different, with Brown (2006) being a bit more conservative.

Sources of Poor Fit

It is not unusual for the initially specified CFA model to fit poorly (or at least not as well as one may wish). Poor fit can result from a number of causes, including specifying too few or too many factors, selecting inappropriate indicators, or defining an incorrect pattern of indicator-factor loadings. In addition, a model may fit poorly because the error theory is incorrectly specified—that is, the model may incorrectly identify measurement errors as uncorrelated or correlated. If the model does not fit well, then the researcher may want to consider revising the model.

Model Revision

If a model does not fit well, the researcher will need to identify the areas of poor fit; then, depending on the areas of poor fit and the indicated revisions, the researcher may modify the model. There are multiple ways to identify areas of poor fit, but changes to the model should only be made when they are consistent with theory or prior research and "make sense." Areas of poor fit can be identified by examination of modification indices and localized areas of strain (i.e., residuals).

Modification Indices

Modification indices (MI) are generated by the software packages; they are data-driven indicators of changes to the model that are likely to improve model fit. MI are analogous to single df χ^2 tests; therefore, an MI greater than 3.84 (or roughly 4) indicates a change that will probably result in a significant improvement in model fit. MI can suggest changes to any aspect of the model, including adding paths between latent variables, adding paths from latent variables to observed variables not originally specified as indicators of that latent variable, adding error covariances between observed variables, and so forth. MI for covariances suggest adding error covariances—either between two errors or between an error and a latent variable. MI for variances suggest adding variances between latent variables. MI for regression weights suggest adding regression paths to the model; for example, suggested paths can be from a latent variable to an observed variable or one observed variable to another. Many of the modifications suggested by the MI may not make sense given theory and prior research; such nonsensical modifications should not be made regardless of how large the parameter change would be.

Localized Areas of Strain

Residuals can be examined to identify localized areas of strain. Standardized residuals greater than 1.96 (for $p < 0.05$) or 2.58 (for $p < 0.01$) may indicate areas of strain. Positive standardized residuals indicate that the model's parameters underestimate the relationship, whereas negative standardized residuals indicate the model's parameters overestimate the relationship.

Specification Search

Once you start modifying a model based on MI or standardized residuals, even if the modifications are justified, you have moved out of the confirmatory framework and into exploratory work. Consequently, respecified models should be interpreted with caution and substantial changes should be replicated in independent samples (MacCallum, 2003), or, if the original study has a sufficiently large sample size, it can be randomly split in half so the initial CFA through model respecification can be conducted on one half of the sample, and then the fit of the final model can be tested in the second half of the sample. MacCallum (2003) suggests that model respecification:

> "should begin with careful review of study design and model specification in search of oversights, alternative designs for evaluating the model of interest, or reasonable alternative or competing models that should be evaluated. . . . one should focus on residual correlations or covariances to identify possible aspects of the model that are not explaining data well and that call for closer examination. Given such information, the model may be modified, or perhaps the study itself re-designed, and a new evaluation of the model conducted. Of critical importance is when a model is modified and eventually found to fit the data well, that model must be validated on new data." (p. 129)

MacCallum (2003) also recommends against the common approach of using modification indices to create a better fitting model because such procedures capitalize on chance and produce unstable results. "Rather than evaluate a single model in isolation, it is often more informative and productive to compare a set of alternative models and possibly select a preferred model from the set" (MacCallum, 2003, p. 130).

Nested Models

Model revision may result in a *nested model* that "contains a subset of the free parameters of another model, which is often referred to as the *parent model*" (Brown, 2006, p. 48). A nested model may result from constraining, rather than freely estimating, some parameters. The χ^2 difference test can be used to test for significance of model improvement with nested models. The χ^2 difference test is conducted by finding the difference between the χ^2 for the parent and nested models (i.e., χ^2 for the parent model minus χ^2 for the nested model) and then finding the difference between the df for the parent and nested models (i.e., df for the parent model minus df for the nested model). The χ^2 difference is then tested for significance for the associated df difference.

For example, if the χ^2 for the parent model equals 246.44 and the χ^2 for the nested model equals 191.07, then the χ^2 difference equals 55.37. If the parent model df equals 74 and the nested model df equals 73, then the df difference equals 1. Using a table of critical values for χ^2, we find that the critical value for a 1 df test is 3.841 (see http://www.itl.nist.gov/div898/handbook/eda/section3/eda3674.htm or almost any introductory statistics book for critical values of the chi-square distribution). Therefore, because our obtained χ^2 difference is greater than 3.841, we can conclude that the change in the model resulted in a significant ($p < 0.05$) improvement in model fit.

Job Satisfaction Scale Confirmatory Factor Analysis Example

We are now going to look at a detailed example of a CFA of the Job Satisfaction Scale (JSS; Koeske, Kirk, Koeske, & Rauktis, 1994) using Amos 7.0 (the raw data can be downloaded from this book's companion Web site). The JSS (Koeske, Kirk, Koeske, & Rauktis, 1994) is a 14-item self-report questionnaire to assess overall satisfaction with employment. As Koeske and colleagues (1994) noted in their introduction, a valid and reliable measure of job satisfaction was needed to advance research and practice in the area of job satisfaction. Much of the prior social work literature approached job satisfaction as a unidimensional factor, rather than as a multidimensional construct with a number of different facets, such as "intrinsic versus extrinsic, interpersonal relations, pay and benefits ... [The JSS is a] brief and direct facet-based measure of job satisfaction among people employed in social services" (Koeske et al., 1994). It is important to note that whereas several theories have been used as the foundation for the job satisfaction construct (van Saane, Sluiter, Verbeek, & Frings-Dresen, 2003), Koeske and colleagues did not provide a specific theoretical foundation for their measure.

Responses on the JSS are measured on a seven-point Likert-type scale ranging from 1 (very dissatisfied) to 7 (very satisfied). Items are categorized into three subscales. *Intrinsic dynamics* include the factors specific to the nature of the work, the type of clients served, and coworker interaction. *Organizational structure* includes the quality of supervision, clarity of job demands, adequacy of funding, and opportunity for employee input. The *salary and promotion* subscale includes items on salary and benefits and the opportunity for advancement.

The JSS yields a full-scale score in addition to the three subscale scores (Koeske & Kelly, 1995). The JSS has adequate reliability and validity and internal consistency reliabilities have been reported between 0.83 and 0.89 for the full scale and subscales (Koeske & Kelly, 1995). For the full JSS scale and the three subscales, higher scores indicate higher levels of job satisfaction.

Factor Structure of the Job Satisfaction Scale

Using an initial merged sample ($n = 159$), "The initial 16-item analysis yielded a four-factor structure, with the fourth factor containing only a single variable or facet (amount of funding for programs). In addition, one item, interpersonal relations with fellow workers, loaded weakly and complexly on the first two factors and had the lowest communally [sic] in the set. Consequently, these two items were dropped, and the data were reanalyzed with a three-factor extraction criterion" (Koeske et al., 1994). Using principal axes extraction with varimax rotation, Koeske et al. reported that all three factors had eigenvalues greater than 1, 53.5% of the common variance was explained, and all final communalities were 0.35 or greater. Oblique rotation did not "markedly alter or improve the solution" (Koeske et al., 1994). These initial analyses were conducted on data collected using an 11-point response scale of −5 (very dissatisfied) to +5 (very satisfied).

The initial 14-item factor structure was partially replicated in a sample of 176 NASW members. However, 3 of the original 14 items were replaced, and a new 7-point response scale was used (1 = very dissatisfied; 7 = very satisfied). However, because the results were somewhat different, a two-factor solution was also tested in both samples. "In general, the two-factor solution produced a good result for both the merged and the NASW samples. 'Chances for acquiring new skills' was the only complex item in both analyses [with loadings of .41 on intrinsic, .29 on organization, and .37 on salary and promotion]. The supervision, salary, and promotion items all loaded on the organization-referring facets, producing a convincing extrinsic job satisfaction (EJS) factor; the IJS [intrinsic job satisfaction] factor remained intact. As might be expected, however, the salary and promotion items had weak loadings on the extrinsic factor in the two-factor solution for the merged sample" (Koeske et al., 1994).

Based on the set of analyses, Koeske et al. (1994) concluded "the 14-item Job Satisfaction Scale is a short, reliable, and valid measure of job satisfaction in the human services. The intrinsic and organization satisfaction subscales can provide more specific information, and we suggest summing the salary and promotion items to provide a third scale. The salary and promotion pair not only split off as a separate factor in most factor analyses, they also relate differently from IJS [intrinsic job satisfaction] and OJS [organizational job satisfaction] to many other variables. An extrinsic score that encompasses OJS and salary and promotion may, nonetheless, be theoretically compatible and suitable in some circumstances." In a later study, a 13-item version of the JSS was used with a three-factor "structure reflecting intrinsic job satisfaction (e.g., challenge of the job, rewards of working with clients), organizational job satisfaction (e.g., amount of authority granted), and extrinsic satisfaction (e.g., salary and benefits)" (Belcastro & Koeske, 1996). Alphas for the intrinsic, organizational, and extrinsic subscales were 0.89, 0.70, and 0.34, respectively; the 13-item scale had an alpha of 0.90. I have provided detailed information about the development and testing of the JSS because the factor analysis findings and their conclusions provide important information for modifications that can be reasonably made in the CFA model that is tested here.

Data for this Example

The data for this example are from a study of U.S. Air Force Family Advocacy Program (FAP) workers (Bean, Harrington, & Pintello, 1998; Harrington, Bean, Pintello, & Mathews, 2001). Based on the Koeske et al. (1994) article, we used the 16-item version of the JSS and the 7-point response set. Item 15 "Your feeling of success as a professional" was changed to "Your feeling of success as a social worker/nurse" to be more applicable for the FAP workers. The sample included 139 FAP workers and the response rate for the survey was 74%. Cronbach's alpha was 0.89 for the 16-item full scale, 0.86 for the 7-item intrinsic subscale, 0.84 for the 5-item organizational subscale, and 0.64 for the 2-item salary/promotion subscale. These are acceptable levels of internal consistency reliability for the full, intrinsic, and organizational scales. The internal consistency reliability for the salary/promotion subscale is a little lower than desirable, and analyses involving this subscale should be interpreted with caution.

Table 4.1 provides a list of the JSS items by subscale, means, medians, skewness, kurtosis, and number of missing cases calculated using SPSS 15.0. The data presented in Table 4.1 are based on all available data (similar to using pairwise deletion), so the sample size varies from 139 for items that all participants answered to a low of 116 for the item that 23 participants did not answer (JSS15).

Data Considerations

As discussed in Chapter 3, there are several important data considerations that need to be addressed, including missing data, normality, and sample size requirements.

Missing Data

As part of preparing data for analysis, it is important to look for missing data. In the FAP dataset, there was some missing data on the JSS. Approximately 80% of the respondents provided valid responses to all 16 JSS items ($n = 110$; 79.1%). Nineteen (13.7%) respondents had missing data on one item, and 10 (7.2%) respondents missed two to five items. Table 4.1 provides the number of respondents who did not answer the item for each JSS item.

As discussed in Chapter 3, there are two recommended options for handling missing data: *(1)* run the analysis with missing data allowing the software to estimate parameters (i.e., direct ML), or *(2)* impute (i.e., use computer software to replace missing values with plausible guesses

Table 4.1 FAP Sample JSS Items, Means, Medians, Skewness, Kurtosis, and Percent Missing ($n = 139$)

Items by Subscale	Mean	Median	Skewness (se skew)	Kurtosis (se kurt)	n and % Missing
Intrinsic Job Satisfaction					
1. Working with your clients.	5.90	6.00	−0.547 (0.209)	−0.773 (0.416)	5 (3.6%)
6. The challenge your job provides you.	5.26	6.00	−1.004 (0.207)	0.248 (0.411)	2 (1.4%)
8. Chances for acquiring new skills.	4.44	5.00	−0.358 (0.206)	−0.775 (0.408)	0 (0%)
9. Amount of client contact.	5.47	6.00	−1.017 (0.208)	0.334 (0.413)	3 (2.2%)
10. Opportunities for really helping people.	5.53	6.00	−1.334 (0.207)	1.729 (0.411)	2 (1.4%)
15. Your feelings of success as a social worker/nurse.	5.39	6.00	−1.152 (0.225)	0.648 (0.446)	23 (16.5%)
16. Field of specialization you are in.	5.42	6.00	−1.046 (0.209)	0.947 (0.414)	4 (2.9%)
Organizational Job Satisfaction					
2. The amount of authority you have been given to do your job.	5.10	6.00	−0.833 (0.206)	−0.463 (0.408)	0 (0%)
7. The quality of supervision you receive.	4.28	5.00	−0.252 (0.206)	−1.446 (0.410)	1 (0.7%)
12. Clarity of guidelines for doing your job.	4.27	5.00	−0.170 (0.207)	−1.219 (.411)	2 (1.4%)
13. Opportunity for involvement in decision-making.	4.78	5.00	−0.597 (0.206)	−0.644 (0.408)	0 (0%)
14. The recognition given your work by your supervisor.	4.32	4.00	−0.277 (0.206)	−1.271 (0.410)	1 (0.7%)
Salary and Promotion Job Satisfaction					
4. Your salary and benefits.	4.75	5.00	−0.569 (0.206)	−0.729 (0.410)	1 (0.7%)
5. Opportunities for promotion.	2.87	2.50	0.641 (0.208)	−0.718 (0.413)	3 (2.2%)
Items Included in JSS Full Scale Score, but not on any Subscales					
3. Interpersonal relations with fellow workers.	4.99	5.00	−0.713 (0.206)	−0.475 (0.408)	0 (0%)
11. Amount of funding for programs.	3.33	3.00	0.274 (0.206)	−1.013 (0.410)	1 (0.7%)

or estimates of what a response might have been) the missing data before running the analysis (Brown, 2006). For the current example, the analyses were first performed on the raw data (i.e., without imputing missing data) in Amos 7.0 using direct ML and estimate means and intercepts, which is an option under *Analysis Properties, Estimation,* to handle the missing data. Because this approach does not include generation of modification indices, we will also impute the missing data and rerun the analysis in Amos 7.0 (this analysis is described later in this chapter).

Normality

Skewness and kurtosis indices are presented in Table 4.1. Following Kline's (2005) suggestion that only variables with skew index absolute values greater than 3 and kurtosis index absolute values greater than 10 are of concern, none of the variables in this analysis has problematic levels of skewness or kurtosis. Therefore, the JSS data appear to be sufficiently univariate normally distributed. By default, Amos 7.0 does not report normality check statistics, and they are not available for data with missing values.

Sample Size

With a sample size of 139 for this example, Kline (2005) would consider this a medium sample size—not so small as to be untenable, but certainly not large either. Given the medium sample size, caution should be used in drawing conclusions, and the possibility of low power should be considered.

Conducting the Confirmatory Factor Analysis in Amos

Figure 4.1 shows the Amos 7.0 Graphics input used to run the initial CFA on the JSS. The Graphics interface in Amos 7.0 is easy to use, and the drawing features are similar to those in Microsoft Word; brief instructions for running a CFA in Amos are provided in Appendix A. One of the advantages of Amos is its relative ease of use, and the graphics interface makes it quite easy to run an analysis if you know what it should look like.

Amos Graphics follows the conventions of structural equation modeling (SEM) diagrams. The ovals represent latent (or unobserved) variables—in this case, *Intrinsic*, *Organizational*, and *Salary/Promotion* represent the three subscales of the JSS. The rectangles represent observed variables, which are the actual JSS items (as listed in Table 4.1). The curved double-headed arrows represent the correlations or covariances among the latent variables (for the standardized and unstandardized solutions, respectively), and the straight single-headed arrows represent the factor loadings of the observed variables on the latent variables. The small circles with arrows pointing from the circles to the observed variables represent errors or unique factors (Arbuckle, 2006b). Notice in Figure 4.1

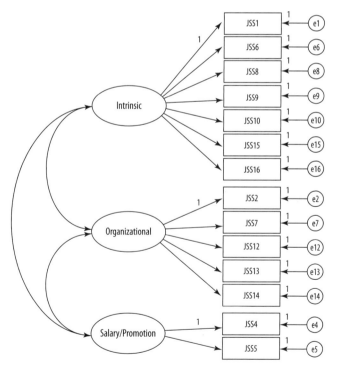

Figure 4.1 JSS CFA Model Amos 7.0 Graphics Input File

that each latent variable has a 1 next to the path from it to one observed variable (e.g., from *Intrinsic* to JSS1). This serves to constrain the parameter and define the scale of the latent variable (Arbuckle, 2006b); each latent variable must be scaled.

Job Satisfaction Scale Confirmatory Factor Analysis Amos 7.0 Output

The standardized estimates output provided by Amos 7.0 using ML estimation with missing data is shown in Figure 4.2. The correlations among the latent variables are shown next to the curved lines. The correlation between *Intrinsic* and *Organizational* is 0.66, the correlation between *Intrinsic* and *Salary/Promotion* is 0.39, and the correlation between *Organizational* and *Salary/Promotion* is 0.49. These correlations suggest that the latent variables are somewhat related, as would be expected given that they are all hypothesized to be aspects of job satisfaction, but the correlations are not so high as to suggest that they are all measuring the same construct. The factor loadings are shown on the arrows from the latent variables to the observed variables. The loadings for the seven variables on *Intrinsic* range from 0.47 (JSS8) to 0.83 (JSS10 and JSS15). The loadings for the five variables on *Organizational* range from 0.56 (JSS12) to 0.80 (JSS13), and the loadings for the two variables on *Salary/Promotion* are 0.54 (JSS4) and 0.94 (JSS5). All loadings and correlations among the latent variables are significant ($p < 0.05$) and all are 0.47 or greater. Using the rules of thumb (Tabachnick & Fidell, 2007) presented in Chapter 2, all the factor loadings are considered fair to excellent, and all indicator variables significantly load on the expected latent variable.

The numbers at the upper right hand corner of each observed variable are the squared multiple correlations for each observed variable. For example, the squared multiple correlation for JSS1 is 0.35, which indicates that 35% of the variance in JSS1 is accounted for by *Intrinsic* and "is an estimate of the lower bound on the reliability" (Arbuckle, 2006b, p. 148) for this item. The remaining 65% of the variance in JSS1 is accounted for by the unique factor e1, which represents the unique aspects of the item or measurement error. The squared multiple correlations for the JSS items range from 0.22 for JSS8 to 0.88 for JSS5.

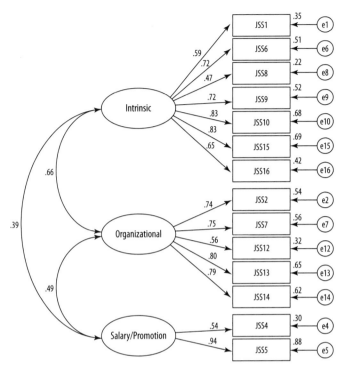

Figure 4.2 FAP Sample JSS CFA Model Standardized Estimates ($n = 139$)

Model Fit

The initial three-factor JSS CFA model did not fit well, with $\chi^2 = 221.875$, $df = 74$, and p less than 0.0005. For this example, all fit indices provided by Amos 7.0 are shown in Table 4.2. In addition to the fit indices recommended by Brown (2006), Amos provides a number of additional fit indices that you may see in the literature; although not all fit indices are recommended, different journals may have different reporting requirements. Using Brown's (2006) recommendations of RMSEA close to 0.06 or less; CFI close to 0.95 or greater; and TLI close to 0.95 or greater, we see that this model does not fit well, with RMSEA = 0.120, CFI = 0.827, and TLI = 0.755. These fit indices suggest that the model needs to be modified.

Table 4.2 FAP Sample Three-Factor JSS CFA Model Fit Summary ($n = 139$)
(Amos 7.0 Output)

CMIN

Model	NPAR	CMIN	DF	p	CMIN/DF
Default model	45	221.875	74	0.000	2.998
Saturated model	119	0.000	0		
Independence model	14	959.792	105	0.000	9.141

Baseline Comparisons

Model	NFI Delta1	RFI rho1	IFI Delta2	TLI rho2	CFI
Default model	0.769	0.672	0.833	0.755	.827
Saturated model	1.000		1.000		1.000
Independence model	0.000	0.000	0.000	0.000	0.000

Parsimony-Adjusted Measures

Model	p-RATIO	p-NFI	p-CFI
Default model	.705	.542	.583
Saturated model	.000	.000	.000
Independence model	1.000	.000	.000

NCP

Model	NCP	LO 90	HI 90
Default model	147.875	106.907	196.476
Saturated model	0.000	0.000	0.000
Independence model	854.792	759.389	957.645

FMIN

Model	FMIN	F0	LO 90	HI 90
Default model	1.608	1.072	0.775	1.424
Saturated model	0.000	0.000	0.000	0.000
Independence model	6.955	6.194	5.503	6.939

RMSEA

Model	RMSEA	LO 90	HI 90	p-CLOSE
Default model	.120	.102	.139	.000
Independence model	.243	.229	.257	.000

AIC

Model	AIC	BCC	BIC	CAIC
Default model	311.875	322.851		
Saturated model	238.000	267.024		
Independence model	987.792	991.207		

(*continued*)

Table 4.2 FAP Sample Three-Factor JSS CFA Model Fit Summary ($n = 139$) (Amos 7.0 Output) (*continued*)

ECVI

Model	ECVI	LO 90	HI 90	MECVI
Default model	2.260	1.963	2.612	2.339
Saturated model	1.725	1.725	1.725	1.935
Independence model	7.158	6.467	7.903	7.183

HOELTER

Model	HOELTER .05	HOELTER .01
Default model	60	66
Independence model	19	21

Multiple models (i.e., default, saturated, and independence) are shown for many of the fit indices. The *default model* is the model specified by the user, so this will provide the fit indices for the model you are testing. The *saturated model* is the most general model possible without any constraints; "it is a vacuous model in the sense that it is guaranteed to fit any set of data perfectly. Any Amos model is a constrained version of the saturated model" (Amos 7.0 Reference Guide Appendix C: Measures of Fit). The *independence model* is the opposite extreme of the saturated model and "is so severely constrained that you would expect it to provide a very poor fit to any interesting set of data. It frequently happens that each one of the models that you have specified can be so constrained as to be equivalent to the independence model" (Amos 7.0 Reference Guide Appendix C: Measures of Fit). Finally, a *zero model* is available for all estimation methods except ML; in this model, all parameters are fixed at zero (the zero model is not shown in Table 4.2 because ML estimation was used for this model).

One of the nice features of Amos 7.0 is that many headings in the Text Output shown in Table 4.2 are hyperlinks, and clicking on them will open a box that describes the fit index and provides additional information about it. For example, clicking on RMSEA will produce the information box shown in Figure 4.3; notice that the definitions for RMSEA and the confidence interval (labeled LO 90 and HI 90), a relevant reference, and a rule of thumb for interpretation are provided.

RMSEA

F_0 incorporates no penalty for model complexity and will tend to favor models with many parameters. In comparing two nested models, F_0 will never favor the simpler model. Steiger and Lind (1980) suggested compensating for the effect of model complexity by dividing F_0 by the number of degrees of freedom for testing the model. Taking the square root of the resulting ratio gives the population "root mean square error of approximation", called RMS by Steiger and Lind, and RMSEA by Browne and Cudeck (1993).

$$\text{population RMSEA} = \sqrt{\frac{F_0}{d}}$$

$$\text{estimated RMSEA} = \sqrt{\frac{\hat{F}_0}{d}}$$

The columns labeled **LO 90** and **HI 90** contain the lower limit and upper limit of a 90% confidence interval for the population value of **RMSEA**. The limits are given by

$$\text{LO } 90 = \sqrt{\frac{\delta_L / n}{d}}$$

$$\text{HI } 90 = \sqrt{\frac{\delta_U / n}{d}}$$

Rule of thumb:

"Practical experience has made us feel that a value of the RMSEA of about .05 or less would indicate a close fit of the model in relation to the degrees of freedom. This figure is based on subjective judgment. It cannot be regarded as infallible or correct, but it is more reasonable than the requirement of exact fit with the RMSEA = 0.0. We are also of the opinion that a value of about 0.08 or less for the RMSEA would indicate a reasonable error of approximation and would not want to employ a model with a RMSEA greater than 0.1." (Browne and Cudeck, 1993)

Use the **\rmsea** text macro to display **RMSEA** on a path diagram. Use **\rmsealo** and **\rmseahi** to display the lower and upper limits of the 90% confidence interval.

Figure 4.3 Amos 7.0 Information Box for RMSEA in Text Output Model Fit Summary Table

Missing Data and Model Modification

Because the initial model does not fit well, we may want to consider modifications, which can be based on modification indices (MI) or examination of residuals. At this point, we still have incomplete data, therefore MI are not available in Amos 7.0. As discussed earlier, prior research and theory are important considerations for specifying a CFA model. However, although the prior work with the JSS suggests some possible modifications, MI would also be helpful.

To examine the MI, SPSS missing values analysis (MVA) using the expectation maximization algorithm was used to impute missing data for the FAP sample. It is important to note that Brown (2006) indicates that this approach has limitations and may result in inconsistent standard errors and, consequently, compromised confidence intervals and significance tests; however, other authors (e.g., Schafer & Graham, 2002) recommend this approach. After running the MVA to impute missing data, we have a "complete" data set because all missing values have been replaced with plausible values. We can now use Amos to generate MI. Figure 4.4 shows the standardized output from Amos 7.0 for the FAP sample with imputed missing data.

As can be seen by comparing Figures 4.2 and 4.4, the standardized estimates are very similar before and after imputing the missing data. Similarly to the original model, this model does not fit well, with RMSEA = 0.130, CFI = 0.821, and TLI = 0.780. (Imputing missing data should not result in extremely different parameter estimates or fit indices, and it is important to compare the analyses conducted both ways. If there are major differences between the analyses, then more work is needed to examine the missing data patterns.) However, in Amos 7.0, this model differs from the original in that we can now obtain an assessment of normality and MI (see Tables 4.3 and 4.4, respectively).

Normality Check

An additional benefit of having a data set without missing data in Amos 7.0 is that you can obtain normality checks, including skewness and kurtosis indexes (as shown in Table 4.3). Mardia's coefficient is a test

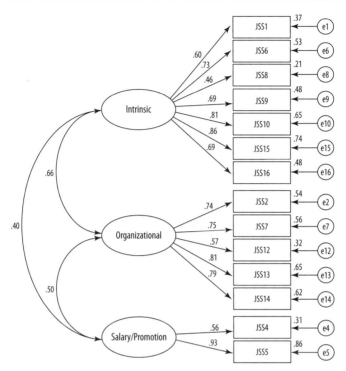

Figure 4.4 FAP Sample JSS With Imputed Missing Data CFA Model Standardized Estimates (*n* = 139)

of multivariate normality—specifically kurtosis—available in Amos. In Table 4.3, Mardia's coefficient is equal to 40.328, and its critical ratio is equal to 11.232. In Amos 7.0, the critical ratio for Mardia's coefficient is equal to Mardia's coefficient divided by its standard error; "assuming normality in very large samples, each of the critical values shown in the table [i.e. Table 4.3] … is an observation on a standard normally distributed random variable" (Amos 7.0 Discussion of NormalityCheck example). In other words, the critical ratio can be interpreted as a *z*-score. It is very important to note that the Amos 7.0 help information reports that this information is of limited use, and it is only of any use when one knows how robust to non-normality the chosen estimation procedure is. Using the criteria provided by Kline (2005), skewness and kurtosis do not appear to be problematic for this example.

Table 4.3 Amos Output Assessment of Normality for FAP JSS Model With Imputed Data ($n = 139$)

Assessment of Normality (Group Number 1)

Variable	min	max	skew	c.r.	kurtosis	c.r.
JSS5	0.741	7.000	0.607	2.921	−0.786	−1.890
JSS4	1.000	7.000	−0.552	−2.657	−0.748	−1.799
JSS14	1.000	7.000	−0.260	−1.254	−1.272	−3.062
JSS13	1.000	7.000	−0.591	−2.843	−0.663	−1.597
JSS12	1.000	7.000	−0.170	−0.821	−1.215	−2.925
JSS7	1.000	7.000	−0.262	−1.262	−1.433	−3.449
JSS2	1.000	7.000	−0.824	−3.968	−0.489	−1.178
JSS16	1.000	7.000	−1.000	−4.812	0.761	1.831
JSS15	0.670	7.000	−1.025	−4.934	0.380	0.913
JSS10	1.000	7.000	−1.258	−6.057	1.352	3.253
JSS9	1.000	7.000	−0.991	−4.772	0.213	0.514
JSS8	1.000	7.000	−0.354	−1.705	−0.790	−1.901
JSS6	1.000	7.000	−0.982	−4.725	0.199	0.479
JSS1	3.000	7.000	−0.547	−2.631	−0.758	−1.824
Multivariate					40.328	11.232

c.r.= critical ratio

Modification Indices

The MI generated by Amos include the actual MI estimate (e.g., 6.682 for adding a covariance between e13 and e5) and Par Change, which is the estimated parameter change that would be obtained if this change were made to the model. Changes made to the model based on MI are data-driven, and as such, making changes based on the MI moves the researcher from the realm of confirmatory analysis into exploratory analysis. However, with that caution in mind, it can be helpful to examine MI for ways to improve model fit and for possible directions for future research. Because the JSS CFA model does not fit well, it seems reasonable to explore ways of possibly improving model fit.

Examining the MI in Table 4.4, two things stand out. First, the largest MI suggests adding a covariance between the errors for JSS9 and JSS10, which allows the model to include an estimate of the amount of relationship between these two errors. Job Satisfaction Scale item 9 is amount of contact with clients and JSS10 is opportunity for really helping people;

both are part of the *Intrinsic* factor. It makes sense that the amount of contact a professional has with clients would be related to opportunities for helping people, in which case adding the covariance between these two errors may be reasonable. (It is important to note that one can almost always come up with a justification for why two error terms could be related and one should be cautious about stretching this logic too far.) The second thing that is apparent from the MI is that several of them involve JSS8, and this item in particular seems to be related to all three factors. From the earlier discussion of the development of the JSS, we know that Koeske and colleagues (1994) found that item 8 was complex and had loadings on all three factors. Given their finding, it is not surprising that there are a number of MI associated with JSS8. Specifically, the MI suggest adding paths from *Salary/Promotion* and *Organizational* to JSS8 (MI of 10.615 and 8.696, respectively). In addition, the MI suggest adding paths between JSS8 and five other variables (JSS5, JSS6, JSS7, JSS13, and JSS14). Finally, the MI suggest adding covariances between the error for JSS8 and all three latent variables and three other errors (e5, e6, and e13). This pattern may either suggest allowing this item to be related to all three factors or dropping it.

Because examination of the MI suggests two primary changes to the model, we will examine the impact of both. First, we will add a covariance between e9 and e10, meaning that we will allow the errors for items JSS9 and JSS10 to be correlated or covary. This results in a nested model (the parent model is the one reported in Figure 4.2) with $\chi^2 = 191.072$ and $df = 73$. Comparing this with the parent model, which had $\chi^2 = 221.875$ and $df = 74$, we can use the χ^2 difference test to determine whether the change to the model results in a significant improvement. The difference between χ^2 for the two models is $221.875 - 191.072 = 30.803$, $df = 1$, p less than 0.0005, indicating that adding the covariance between the errors for JSS9 and JSS10 results in an improvement in the model. Other fit indices also show some improvement in model fit (RMSEA = 0.108, CFI = 0.878, and TLI = 0.847); however, the model still does not fit well.

Examining the MI for this modified model, we see that several of the suggested modifications still involve JSS8, including adding paths from *Organizational* and *Salary/Promotion* to JSS8, and adding paths between

Table 4.4 Amos Selected Output Modification Indices for FAP JSS Model With Imputed Data ($n = 139$)

Covariances: (Group Number 1—Default Model)

			Modification Index	Par Change
e13	↔	e5	6.682	0.392
e7	↔	e14	6.679	0.497
e16	↔	e4	7.020	0.393
e16	↔	e13	4.124	−0.230
e15	↔	e4	4.881	0.286
e15	↔	e13	4.432	0.209
e15	↔	e16	15.495	0.355
e10	↔	e4	4.051	−0.262
e10	↔	e16	14.870	−0.352
e9	↔	Salary/Promotion	7.576	−0.267
e9	↔	e13	6.104	−0.292
e9	↔	e12	6.016	0.376
e9	↔	e16	10.616	−0.355
e9	↔	e15	9.667	−0.292
e9	↔	e10	46.201	0.647
e8	↔	Salary/Promotion	6.104	0.330
e8	↔	Organizational	10.387	0.514
e8	↔	Intrinsic	9.251	−0.224
e8	↔	e5	10.185	0.645
e8	↔	e13	9.886	0.512
e6	↔	Salary/Promotion	6.856	0.262
e6	↔	e5	10.284	0.486
e6	↔	e12	17.750	−0.666
e6	↔	e8	5.614	0.384
e1	↔	e16	6.284	0.205

Regression Weights: (Group Number 1—Default Model)

			Modification Index	Par Change
JSS5	←	JSS8	7.396	0.194
JSS4	←	JSS16	4.058	0.183
JSS13	←	JSS8	8.548	0.168
JSS12	←	JSS6	6.719	−0.209
JSS16	←	JSS4	6.821	0.135
JSS16	←	JSS10	4.293	−0.131
JSS16	←	JSS9	5.052	−0.139
JSS15	←	JSS4	4.288	0.093
JSS15	←	JSS13	4.300	0.096
JSS15	←	JSS16	7.636	0.156

(*continued*)

Table 4.4   Amos Selected Output Modification Indices for FAP JSS Model With Imputed Data (*n* = 139) (*continued*)

Regression Weights: (Group Number 1—Default Model)

			Modification Index	Par Change
JSS15	←	JSS9	4.732	−0.117
JSS10	←	JSS4	6.273	−0.113
JSS10	←	JSS16	7.216	−0.152
JSS10	←	JSS9	22.265	0.255
JSS9	←	Salary/Promotion	6.907	−0.272
JSS9	←	JSS5	6.529	−0.135
JSS9	←	JSS4	6.917	−0.142
JSS9	←	JSS16	5.089	−0.152
JSS9	←	JSS10	13.341	0.241
JSS8	←	Salary/Promotion	10.615	0.464
JSS8	←	Organizational	8.696	0.304
JSS8	←	JSS5	11.488	0.246
JSS8	←	JSS14	8.796	0.193
JSS8	←	JSS13	14.975	0.295
JSS8	←	JSS7	5.537	0.143
JSS6	←	JSS5	5.047	0.122
JSS6	←	JSS12	13.526	−0.204
JSS6	←	JSS8	4.306	0.119

all three latent variables and the error term for JSS8. Given this pattern and Koeske and colleagues' (1994) finding that JSS8 was a complex item, we will try omitting this variable from the model. This second modification results in the following fit indices: χ^2 = 148.030 and *df* = 61, RMSEA = 0.102, CFI = 0.904, and TLI = 0.877. Although this model still does not reach the guidelines provided by Brown (2006), the model fits noticeably better than the earlier two models.

Finally, examining the MI for this second modified model, there are now many fewer MI reported and most are smaller than in the initial model (see Table 4.5). The largest remaining MI suggest adding error covariances between e6 and e12 (MI = 13.976) and e5 and e6 (MI = 10.626). JSS5 is "opportunities for promotion" (on the *Salary/Promotion* factor), JSS6 is "the challenge your job provides you" (on the *Intrinsic* factor), and JSS12 is "clarity of guidelines for doing your job" (on the *Organizational* factor). One could argue that all three items may reflect constraints put on professionals by the organization in which they are employed, which would suggest that it might be reasonable to add covariances between e6 and e12 and between e6 and e5. (At this point, we are clearly into data-driven changes, and as such the modified model would need to be replicated!)

The final version of the JSS model retains the original three-factor structure but drops item 8 and adds three error covariances between the error terms for items 9 and 10, items 6 and 12, and items 5 and 6. The Amos Graphics final modified model is shown in Figure 4.5, and the standardized output is shown in Figure 4.6. This third and final modification

Table 4.5 Amos Selected Output Modification Indices for FAP JSS Model With Imputed Data After Making Modifications 1 and 2 ($n = 139$)

Covariances: (Group Number 1—Default Model)

			Modification Index	Par Change
e13	↔	e5	6.891	0.399
e7	↔	e14	7.057	0.514
e16	↔	Organizational	5.765	−0.254
e16	↔	e4	5.014	0.312
e16	↔	e13	6.870	−0.279
e15	↔	e13	4.496	0.197
e10	↔	e16	6.066	−0.177
e9	↔	e13	5.052	−0.223
e6	↔	Salary/Promotion	5.141	0.247
e6	↔	e5	10.626	0.508
e6	↔	e4	4.028	−0.328
e6	↔	e12	13.976	−0.607
e1	↔	e16	5.417	0.182
e1	↔	e9	8.422	0.211

Regression Weights: (Group Number 1—Default Model)

			Modification Index	Par Change
JSS12	←	JSS6	6.397	−0.204
JSS16	←	JSS4	4.114	0.098
JSS16	←	JSS13	5.918	−0.121
JSS16	←	JSS10	4.438	−0.125
JSS9	←	JSS1	5.290	0.180
JSS6	←	JSS5	4.967	0.124
JSS6	←	JSS12	9.699	−0.177
JSS1	←	JSS9	5.469	0.114

results in the following fit indices: $\chi^2 = 125.049$, $df = 59$, RMSEA = 0.090, CFI = 0.927, and TLI = 0.903. Using Brown's (2006) recommendations of RMSEA close to 0.06 or less, CFI close to 0.95 or greater, and TLI close to 0.95 or greater, we see that this model does not fit perfectly, but it comes much closer to the recommended levels than the previous models.

This sequence of modifications has resulted in a better fitting model, and whereas the changes seem plausible given the findings reported by Koeske et al. (1994), the changes are primarily data-driven, and as such the model should be tested in an independent sample, which we will do in the Chapter 5. Two other general comments about this CFA example: First, the *Salary/Promotion* subscale only has two items, which may contribute to the moderate fit of this model. In general, models should have at least three indicators for each latent variable. Second, there are several

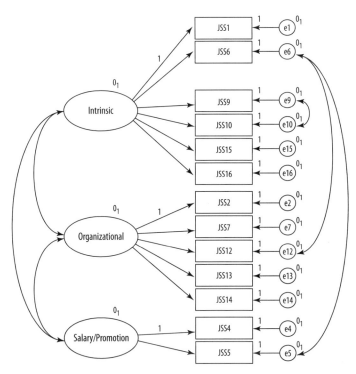

Figure 4.5 JSS CFA Model With Three Modifications (Final Model) From Amos 7.0 Graphics

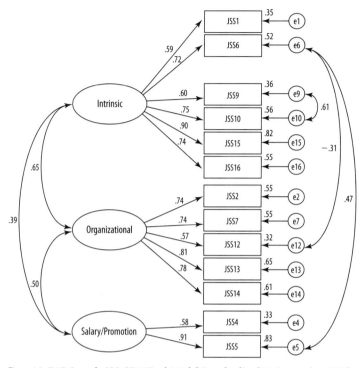

Figure 4.6 FAP Sample JSS CFA Final Model Standardized Estimates ($n = 139$)

limitations to this analysis, including the moderate sample size and modifications made to one of the items for the original study. Therefore, the findings should be interpreted cautiously and *not* taken as an indication of problems or limitations with the JSS.

Chapter Summary

This chapter examined assessing CFA model fit and model revision. Assessment of model fit involves considering a number of indices of model fit; fit indices were grouped into categories of absolute fit, parsimony correction, comparative fit, and predictive fit. Recommendations for identifying acceptable model fit were presented, and methods of finding sources of poor fit were discussed. Model revision, including the use and testing of nested models, modification indices, localized areas of strain, and specification search, was discussed. A detailed CFA example using JSS data was presented, and each aspect of conducting a CFA, including prior research and theory, data considerations, conducting the CFA in Amos 7.0, model fit, and model modification, was addressed.

Suggestions for Further Reading

See Arbuckle (2006b) and Byrne (2001a) for much more information on how to use Amos 7.0 Graphics.

5

Use of Confirmatory Factor Analysis with Multiple Groups

This chapter will focus on using multiple-group confirmatory factor analysis (CFA) to examine the appropriateness of CFA models across different groups and populations (multiple-group CFA across time will be briefly discussed in Chapter 6). Two examples of multiple-group CFA from the social work literature will be discussed, and then we will present a detailed multiple-group CFA building on the Job Satisfaction Scale (JSS) example presented in the Chapter 5. Please note that this is one of the more complex uses of CFA, and this chapter is intended to briefly introduce this topic; interested readers should examine other resources provided at the end of the chapter for more information.

Multiple Group Confirmatory Factor Analysis

One of the major advantages of CFA is the ability to examine the equivalence of the measurement and structural models across multiple groups (Brown, 2006). The measurement model includes the measurement characteristics of the observed measures, including the factor loadings, intercepts, and residual variances. The structural model includes the latent variables and their factor variances, covariances, and latent means.

In addition, multiple-group CFA compares groups within the latent variable measurement model context, adjusting for measurement errors, correlated residuals, and so forth. Multiple-group CFA involves simultaneous CFAs in two or more groups, using separate variance–covariance matrices (or raw data) for each group. The equivalence or invariance of measurement can be tested by placing equality constraints on parameters in the groups. Equality constraints require parts of the model to be equivalent across groups; they will be discussed in detail and will be used in a data example later in this chapter.

Considerations for Conducting a Multiple-Group Confirmatory Factor Analysis

Several factors may affect the appropriateness of conducting a multiple-group CFA. As discussed in Chapter 3, CFA requires relatively large samples. Several aspects of CFA testing (e.g., the χ^2 difference test) are dependent on sample size, so equal or similar size groups will make interpretation easier. However, multiple-group CFA does not require equal sample sizes in each group and can be performed with unequal group sizes. If unequal groups are be used, then interpretation of the results should consider this issue (Brown, 2006).

Partial measurement invariance is a second consideration, where invariance is present for some, but not all, parameters (Brown, 2006). Byrne (2001a) suggests that partial measurement invariance complicates testing further invariance but that it can still be performed. Allowing for partial measurement invariance can be "very helpful in cases where the evaluation of structural parameters is of greatest substantive interest" (Brown, 2006, p. 300). There are currently no guidelines for how much invariance is acceptable. Moreover, analyses with partial invariance are exploratory and may capitalize on chance, and therefore, they should be interpreted with caution, and findings should be cross-validated if possible (Brown, 2006).

Marker variable selection (i.e., scaling the latent variable, as discussed in Chapter 2) is a third consideration. Marker variable selection is always an important consideration, but it is even more important in multiple-group CFA, where selection of a marker variable that is not invariant across groups could result in poor fit indices and tests of partial invariance.

Brown (2006) suggests running the multiple-group CFA several times with different marker indicators each time. A final consideration involves the use of the χ^2 difference test. As discussed in Chapter 4, there are multiple fit indices that are recommended for testing the goodness of fit of CFA models. Although χ^2 is used for testing nested models, it is not generally recommended for testing the overall fit of a model because of its dependence on sample size. However, even with this limitation, the χ^2 statistic is used for testing invariance across multiple groups. Because of the sensitivity to sample size for χ^2, it is possible to have a significant χ^2 test but not be able to identify any areas of strain in the model where constraints should be relaxed, suggesting that the significant χ^2 is detecting trivial changes without any substantive importance (Brown, 2006, p. 303).

Steps in Conducting a Multiple-Group Confirmatory Factor Analysis

In its strictest sense, a multiple-group CFA would be fully constrained so that all parts of the model have to be exactly equal in all groups. There are two basic ways that this can be tested. The first method would be to start by testing the fully constrained multiple-group CFA model and then relax constraints if the fully constrained model does not fit well. The potential difficulty with this approach is that if the fully constrained model does not fit well, it can be difficult to isolate the parts of the model that need to have the constraints relaxed. The second approach is to build from the least constrained to a fully constrained multiple-group CFA model. Using this approach may involve more steps if the fully constrained model ultimately fits well, but given that this is far from guaranteed, the extra steps will make it easier to identify the parts of the model that are not equivalent across groups.

Brown (2006, pp. 269–270) recommends the following steps for testing a multiple-group CFA:

1. Test the CFA model separately in each group.
2. Conduct the simultaneous test of equal form (identical factor structure).

3. Test the equality of factor loadings.
4. Test the equality of indicator intercepts.
5. Test the equality of indicator residual variances (optional).
6. Test the equality of factor variances.
7. Test the equality of factor covariances (if applicable—that is, there is more than one latent factor).
8. Test the equality of latent means.

The first five steps test measurement invariance; the fifth step of testing the equality of indicator residual variances is optional because it rarely holds in real data and is highly restrictive (Brown, 2006). However, this condition is less important than the first four steps. Steps six through eight test population heterogeneity and would only be tested if that is of interest. Because constrained models are nested within less constrained models, the χ^2 difference test can be used to test whether adding constraints significantly changes the fit of the model.

Equality Constraints

The different parameters that can be estimated in a CFA model were briefly introduced in Chapter 2. There are three types of parameters: *(1)* freely estimated, *(2)* fixed, and *(3)* constrained. *Freely estimated,* or *"free,"* parameters are unknowns that are estimated by the analysis. The analysis will find the best value for each freely estimated parameter that together with other model estimates, will minimize "the differences between the observed and predicted variance-covariance matrices" (Brown, 2006, p. 237). *Fixed* parameters are set to a specific value by the researcher. For example, in Chapter 2 we discussed scaling the latent variable, which is often done by setting or fixing the factor loading for one indicator to "1" so that the latent variable will be scaled (i.e., have the same unit of measurement) to that indicator. Another example of a fixed parameter is when we do not estimate error covariances in a model, in which case the error covariances are set or fixed to 0. *Constrained* parameters are unknowns, like free parameters, but in this case, the parameters are not free to be any value because they have been constrained or restricted to certain values. *Equality constraints* force the unstandardized parameters to be equal; these are the most common type of constrained parameters (Brown, 2006, p. 237).

It is important to note that the constraints are placed on the *unstandardized* solution and the constrained parameters must have the same metric. For example, on the JSS, all the items are measured on the same Likert-type scale, so they have the same metric, and it would be possible to constrain the factor loadings to be equal for all items that load on one latent variable. However, if we had indicators measured on different metrics (e.g., some on a 7-point Likert-type scale and others on a 1-to-100 scale), then it would not be appropriate to constrain the parameters to be equal. Models with equality constraints are nested models, and therefore χ^2 difference testing can be used to statistically compare the models (Brown, 2006).

There are just a few more pertinent definitions to cover before we turn to the specifics of multiple-group CFA. *Congeneric indicators* are expected to measure the same construct, but their measurement errors are independent and their factor loadings and measurement errors are free to vary (Brown, 2006). The CFA model presented in Figure 2.1 is an example of a congeneric model. Note that congeneric indicators load on only one latent variable.

There are two more restrictive types of models. *Tau-equivalent* models have "a congeneric solution in which the indicators of a given factor have equal loadings but differing error variances" (Brown, 2006, p. 239). If Figure 2.1 were tau-equivalent, observed variables 1, 2, and 3 would have equal loadings on latent variable 1, and observed variables 4, 5, and 6 would have equal loadings on latent variable 2; error variances would be allowed to differ. Models with *parallel indicators* have the most restrictions, requiring equal loadings and equal error variances, meaning that "parallel indicators are assumed to measure the latent construct with the same level of precision (i.e., reflected by equivalent error variances)" (Brown, 2006, p. 239). If Figure 2.1 were a parallel model, then the observed variables for each latent variable would need to have equal loadings and equal error variances. When indicators are parallel, they are interchangeable indicators of a latent construct (Brown, 2006, p. 247).

Multiple Group Confirmatory Factor Analysis Examples in the Social Work Literature

Several examples of multiple-group CFAs can be found in the social work literature, and readers are encouraged to look for examples in their substantive area of interest. We will briefly review two articles that used multiple-group CFA.

Group Engagement Measure

Macgowan and Newman (2005) examined the factor structure of the Group Engagement Measure across clinical and nonclinical groups. The Group Engagement Measure (Macgowan, 1997, cited in Macgowan & Newman, 2005) was developed as a 37-item scale with seven dimensions based on theory. The sample included 207 adults; data were collected as part of three separate studies, which yielded 125 participants from clinical settings and 82 social work graduate students (i.e., the nonclinical sample). Confirmatory factor analyses were conducted using Amos 4.0.1 with maximum likelihood (ML) estimation. The 37-item model had acceptable fit in the combined sample, but the authors eliminated 10 items to create a shorter version. The 27-item model fit well (Standardized Root Mean Square Residual [SRMR] = 0.05, root mean square error of approximation [RMSEA] = 0.05, comparative fit index [CFI] = 0.95, and factor loadings were all strong).

Although the CFA model fit well in the combined group, minimum fit criteria were not met when the sample was split into the clinical and nonclinical groups. Specifically, minimum fit was not achieved in the nonclinical student group, and a negative error estimate was found for one of the items. Even after deleting the problematic item, fit indices were still unacceptable (CFI = 0.88 and RMSEA = 0.10). The authors then re-examined the factor that included the problematic item and decided that the factor (contracting) may not have the same meaning for the students and clinical group. The revised six-factor model fit well in the combined group, but the model still did not fit adequately in the two separate groups. To achieve adequate fit in both groups, a second factor (attendance) was dropped; the final five-factor model fit adequately across both groups. The authors concluded that separate models of engagement may be needed for clinical and nonclinical groups.

Safe At Home Instrument

The Safe At Home instrument is "a 35-item self-report measure designed for social work assessment of individuals' readiness to change their intimate partner violence behaviors" (Begun et al., 2003, p. 80). Men were recruited from two sources in Milwaukee, Wisconsin (n = 1,247) and Howard County, Maryland (n = 112). An initial exploratory factor analysis (EFA) was conducted on a sample of 829 men from the Milwaukee sample; a three-factor solution (Precontemplation, Contemplation, and Preparation/Action) based on the stages of change model was identified. The eight items with the highest loadings on each of the three factors were selected, resulting in a 24-item scale. Two CFAs were tested for the three eight-item factors identified in the EFA "to determine whether or not the scale structure was consistent (a) across new samples and (b) across intake and postintervention administrations" (Begun et al., 2003, p. 93). The first CFA on intake data included the Howard County sample and 418 men from Milwaukee who were not included in the initial EFA. Post-intervention data from Howard County and Milwaukee were used in the second CFA. Analyses were conducted using LISREL 8.3, with ML estimation.

An additional CFA was conducted to assess measurement invariance across samples from five intervention programs (Begun et al., 2003). Begun and colleagues (2003) noted that "whereas the fit indices change very little when moving from the baseline to the full measurement invariance model, the difference in χ^2 observed across groups is significant. This suggests some lack of measurement invariance" (p. 97). Examination of modification indices suggested that one item loaded differently in the groups, and allowing that one item to have different loadings across the five samples resulted in "only a marginal reduction in fit relative to the baseline model ($p > .015$), suggesting that apart from this item, the test is measurement invariant over the different programs" (p. 97). The authors note that the findings were specific to men who had been violent toward female intimate partners, and additional research was needed with women and for same-sex partners.

Job Satisfaction Scale Multiple-Group Confirmatory Factor Analysis

We will continue to use the JSS data presented in Chapter 4 for a multiple-group CFA example. The second sample is from an Internet survey of social workers; the same 16-item version of the JSS used in the U.S. Air Force Family Advocacy Program (FAP) study was included in the survey. Ninety-eight respondents completed the JSS as part of the larger Internet survey (the data for this example are available at this book's companion Web site). Following Brown's (2006) recommendations, we will begin by conducting the CFA in the two samples separately.

The results of the CFA for the FAP sample were reported in Chapter 4. Briefly, in the FAP sample, the final version of the JSS model retained the original three-factor structure, but dropped item 8 and added three error covariances between the error terms for items 9 and 10, items 6 and 12, and items 5 and 6. The revised model has the following fit indices: $\chi^2 = 125.049$, $df = 59$, RMSEA = 0.090, CFI = 0.927, and Tucker–Lewis index (TLI) = 0.903. Using Brown's (2006) recommendations of RMSEA close to 0.06 or less; CFI close to 0.95 or greater; and TLI close to 0.95 or greater, we see that there is still room for improvement, but the model fits reasonably well.

Internet Sample Job Satisfaction Scale Confirmatory Factor Analysis

Because the modifications needed to produce an adequately fitting model in the FAP sample may have been sample-specific, we will begin by testing the initial JSS three-factor structure in the Internet sample. In Amos 7.0, it is very easy to run the same CFA model on a new sample of data. Open the Amos 7.0 Graphics file used to run the JSS CFA on the FAP sample (shown in Figure 4.1), then click on File, then Data Files, and browse under File Name to find the new data set to be analyzed. (After you have selected the new data set, you may want to save the Amos file to a new name so that you can keep the results from the two samples separate.) Before conducting the CFA, we need to check the normality assumption to determine whether ML estimation can be appropriately used. Because the Internet sample has complete data, the assessment of normality is available in Amos 7.0 and is shown in Table 5.1 for this sample. Following Kline's (2005) recommendations, none of the variables are considered significantly skewed or kurtotic, and ML estimation can be used. The standardized solution for the Internet sample is shown in Figure 5.1, and selected Amos output is presented in Table 5.1. The fit indices for the Internet sample are $\chi^2 = 222.320$, $df = 74$, $\chi^2/df = 3.004$, Root Mean Square Residual (RMR) = 0.223, goodness-of-fit index (GFI) = 0.751, TLI = 0.798, CFI = 0.836, RMSEA = 0.144, 90% confidence interval for RMSEA = 0.122 to 0.166, Akaike information criterion (AIC) = 284.320, and expected cross-validated index (ECVI) = 2.931.

Similarly to the FAP sample JSS CFA, this initial model does not fit well, although all loadings and correlations among the latent variables are significant. Correlations among the latent variables range from 0.48 between *Salary/Promotion* and *Intrinsic* job satisfaction to 0.84 between *Organizational* and *Intrinsic* job satisfaction. Standardized factor loadings range from 0.63 for JSS1 to 0.86 for JSS6 for *Intrinsic* job satisfaction; from 0.63 for JSS7 to 0.86 for JSS2 for *Organizational* satisfaction; and from 0.56 for JSS4 to 0.79 for JSS5 for *Salary/Promotion* satisfaction. The initial model fit for the Internet sample is remarkably similar to the initial model fit for the FAP sample (see Table 4.2).

Internet Sample Model Modification

Because the model does not fit well, we will examine the modification indices (MI) shown in Table 5.1. The pattern of MI for the Internet sample is a bit different than the pattern seen for the FAP sample. In the FAP

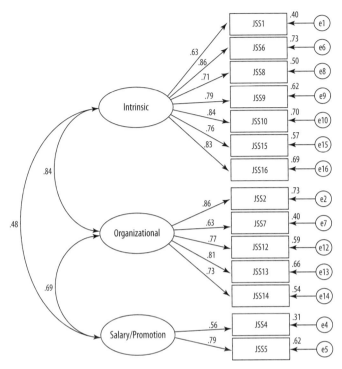

Figure 5.1 Internet Sample JSS CFA Model Standardized Estimates
(n = 98)

sample, examination of the MI suggested two primary changes to the model: *(1)* adding a covariance between e9 and e10, meaning that we will allow the errors for items 9 and 10 to be correlated or covary, and *(2)* dropping JSS8 from the model. Although these changes did not result in an adequately fitting model, fit was noticeably better. After those two modifications, the largest remaining MI suggested adding error covariances between e6 and e12 (MI = 13.976) and e5 and e6 (MI = 10.626), which resulted in a reasonably well fitting model for the FAP sample.

Examining the MI for the Internet sample, we see that the largest MIs are for adding an error covariance between e9 and e14 (MI = 17.373) and adding an error covariance between e1 and e9 (MI = 15.558). (Note that none of the MI for the Internet sample are as large as those found for the FAP sample.) JSS8 again appears to be a complex item, with an MI

Table 5.1 Internet Sample JSS CFA Amos 7.0 Output

Assessment of Normality (Group Number 1)

Variable	Min	Max	Skew	c.r.	Kurtosis	c.r.
JSS5	1.000	7.000	0.051	0.205	−1.047	−2.116
JSS4	1.000	7.000	−0.364	−1.473	−0.888	−1.794
JSS14	1.000	7.000	−0.512	−2.069	−1.007	−2.035
JSS13	1.000	7.000	−0.778	−3.145	−0.461	−0.932
JSS12	1.000	7.000	−0.674	−2.723	−0.376	−0.761
JSS7	1.000	7.000	−0.275	−1.113	−1.108	−2.240
JSS2	1.000	7.000	−1.285	−5.195	1.027	2.075
JSS16	1.000	7.000	−1.549	−6.262	2.939	5.939
JSS15	1.000	7.000	−1.109	−4.480	1.103	2.229
JSS10	1.000	7.000	−1.579	−6.381	1.831	3.701
JSS9	1.000	7.000	−1.221	−4.934	1.116	2.256
JSS8	1.000	7.000	−0.697	−2.818	−0.597	−1.207
JSS6	1.000	7.000	−1.303	−5.267	1.282	2.591
JSS1	1.000	7.000	−1.536	−6.207	2.517	5.086
Multivariate					47.461	11.099

Estimates (Group Number 1—Default Model)
Scalar Estimates (Group Number 1—Default Model)
Maximum Likelihood Estimates
Regression Weights: (Group Number 1—Default Model)

	Estimate	S.E.	C.R.	p	Label
JSS1 ← Intrinsic	1.000				
JSS6 ← Intrinsic	1.567	0.227	6.899	***	par_1
JSS8 ← Intrinsic	1.435	0.240	5.981	***	par_2
JSS10 ← Intrinsic	1.669	0.246	6.786	***	par_3
JSS15 ← Intrinsic	1.315	0.209	6.298	***	par_4
JSS16 ← Intrinsic	1.295	0.192	6.763	***	par_5
JSS2 ← Organizational	1.000				
JSS7 ← Organizational	0.874	0.128	6.821	***	par_6
JSS12 ← Organizational	0.946	0.106	8.931	***	par_7
JSS13 ← Organizational	1.113	0.114	9.761	***	par_8
JSS14 ← Organizational	1.052	0.126	8.330	***	par_9
JSS4 ← Salary/Promotion	1.000				
JSS5 ← Salary/Promotion	1.356	0.356	3.808	***	par_10
JSS9 ← Intrinsic	1.360	0.210	6.490	***	par_11

(*continued*)

Table 5.1 Internet Sample JSS CFA Amos 7.0 Output (*continued*)

Standardized Regression Weights: (Group Number 1—Default Model)

	Estimate
JSS1 ← Intrinsic	.632
JSS6 ← Intrinsic	.855
JSS8 ← Intrinsic	.707
JSS10 ← Intrinsic	.836
JSS15 ← Intrinsic	.756
JSS16 ← Intrinsic	.832
JSS2 ← Organizational	.857
JSS7 ← Organizational	.633
JSS12 ← Organizational	.768
JSS13 ← Organizational	.813
JSS14 ← Organizational	.732
JSS4 ← Salary/Promotion	.558
JSS5 ← Salary/Promotion	.789
JSS9 ← Intrinsic	.786

Covariances: (Group Number 1—Default Model)

	Estimate	S.E.	c.r.	p	Label
Intrinsic ↔ Organizational	0.942	0.204	4.621	***	par_12
Organizational ↔ Salary/ Promotion	0.941	0.285	3.297	***	par_13
Intrinsic ↔ Salary/Promotion	0.396	0.148	2.668	0.008	par_14

Correlations: (Group Number 1—Default Model)

	Estimate
Intrinsic ↔ Organizational	0.840
Organizational ↔ Salary/Promotion	0.686
Intrinsic ↔ Salary/Promotion	0.479

Variances: (Group Number 1—Default Model)

	Estimate	S.E.	c.r.	p	Label
Intrinsic	0.676	0.200	3.379	***	par_15
Organizational	1.863	0.362	5.142	***	par_16
Salary/Promotion	1.009	0.411	2.459	.014	par_17
e1	1.017	0.154	6.622	***	par_18
e6	0.609	0.110	5.545	***	par_19
e8	1.391	0.216	6.448	***	par_20
e9	0.771	0.126	6.124	***	par_21
e10	0.813	0.141	5.760	***	par_22

(*continued*)

Table 5.1 Internet Sample JSS CFA Amos 7.0 Output (*continued*)

	Estimate	S.E.	c.r.	p	Label
e15	0.877	0.140	6.275	***	par_23
e16	0.506	0.087	5.798	***	par_24
e2	0.672	0.132	5.096	***	par_25
e7	2.131	0.327	6.524	***	par_26
e12	1.164	0.194	6.010	***	par_27
e13	1.182	0.209	5.656	***	par_28
e14	1.785	0.288	6.198	***	par_29
e4	2.230	0.397	5.624	***	par_30
e5	1.123	0.459	2.444	0.015	par_31

Squared Multiple Correlations: (Group Number 1—Default Model)

	Estimate
JSS5	.623
JSS4	.312
JSS14	.536
JSS13	.661
JSS12	.589
JSS7	.401
JSS2	.735
JSS16	.692
JSS15	.571
JSS10	.698
JSS9	.619
JSS8	.500
JSS6	.732
JSS1	.399

Modification Indices (Group Number 1—Default Model)
Covariances: (Group Number 1—Default Model)

	Modification Index	Par Change
e14 ↔ Intrinsic	4.435	−0.165
e13 ↔ Organizational	4.294	0.206
e13 ↔ Intrinsic	8.257	−0.189
e13 ↔ e14	11.494	0.571
e7 ↔ e14	11.935	0.740
e7 ↔ e13	4.103	−0.366
e7 ↔ e12	8.373	0.507
e2 ↔ Intrinsic	6.017	0.125
e2 ↔ e14	5.736	−.316
e2 ↔ e13	4.033	0.221

(*continued*)

Table 5.1 Internet Sample JSS CFA Amos 7.0 Output (*continued*)

	Modification Index	Par Change
e2 ↔ e7	5.473	−0.332
e15 ↔ e14	11.638	0.479
e10 ↔ e2	10.324	0.301
e9 ↔ e14	17.373	−0.555
e9 ↔ e13	4.533	−0.240
e9 ↔ e12	7.389	0.296
e9 ↔ e10	5.186	0.209
e8 ↔ Salary/Promotion	9.618	0.397
e8 ↔ Intrinsic	4.392	−0.143
e8 ↔ e5	9.095	0.526
e8 ↔ e16	4.009	−0.191
e6 ↔ Salary/Promotion	9.132	0.274
e6 ↔ e4	7.118	0.373
e6 ↔ e8	7.934	0.300
e1 ↔ e14	5.442	−0.344
e1 ↔ e15	10.123	−0.327
e1 ↔ e9	15.558	0.384

Regression Weights: (Group Number 1—Default Model)

	Modification Index	Par Change
JSS14 ← JSS4	4.554	0.169
JSS14 ← JSS7	6.790	0.197
JSS14 ← JSS9	10.767	−0.330
JSS14 ← JSS1	6.013	−0.269
JSS13 ← JSS14	4.910	0.137
JSS13 ← JSS9	5.172	−0.193
JSS12 ← JSS7	4.772	0.135
JSS12 ← JSS9	5.252	0.188
JSS7 ← JSS14	5.022	0.174
JSS2 ← JSS10	6.788	0.151
JSS15 ← JSS14	6.072	0.125
JSS15 ← JSS1	5.831	−0.185
JSS9 ← JSS14	10.383	−0.155
JSS9 ← JSS1	8.972	0.218
JSS8 ← Salary/Promotion	11.354	0.484
JSS8 ← JSS5	13.563	0.265
JSS6 ← JSS4	8.765	0.145
JSS1 ← JSS9	5.306	0.170

suggestive of allowing it to load on the *Salary/Promotion* latent variable, and MIs suggesting e8 is related to both the *Salary/Promotion* and *Intrinsic* latent variables. Although there are larger MI for this sample, given the earlier discussion of item JSS8 and its complex loadings on all three factors, it seems reasonable to try dropping that variable from the analysis as the first modification. The fit indices for the Internet sample three-factor model without JSS8 are χ^2 = 190.877, *df* = 62, χ^2/df = 3.079, RMR = 0.210, GFI = 0.770, TLI = 0.803, CFI = 0.844, RMSEA = 0.146, 90% confidence interval for RMSEA = 0.123 to 0.170, AIC = 248.877, and ECVI = 2.566. Again the fit indices are lower than desired, but because the MI found for this analysis suggest adding error covariances that were not found for the FAP sample (e.g., error covariance between e9 and e14; MI = 16.511), we will try fitting the multiple groups CFA for the JSS rather than proceeding with changes based on the Internet sample analysis MI.

Multiple-Group Analysis for Job Satisfaction Scale

To run the multiple groups analysis in Amos 7.0 Graphics, the model will be built the same way it was for the one-group CFA models (i.e., as shown in Figure 4.1), and the data for the two samples can be held in two separate data files. The appropriate data files for each group are identified under File, Data Files. Because of the known complexity of JSS8 and given that dropping it from both of the single-group confirmatory factor analyses resulted in improved model fit, we will run the multiple-group CFA on the three-factor model without JSS8. The model to be tested is shown in Figure 5.2 and has six items on the *Intrinsic* latent factor, five items on the *Organizational* latent factor, and two items on the *Salary/Promotion* latent factor. (Note the labels for each parameter in Figure 5.2, such as ccc1_2 for the covariance between *Intrinsic* and *Organizational*, are added by Amos 7.0 when running a multiple-group CFA.)

In Amos 7.0 Graphics, you can test equality constraints by clicking on Analyze, then Multiple-Group Analysis. A message box will pop up that says "The program will remove any models that you have added to the list

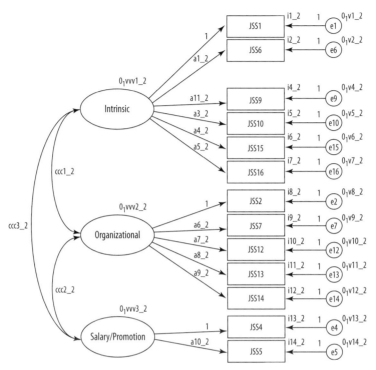

Figure 5.2 Amos 7.0 Graphics Model for Running the Multiple-Group CFA on the JSS for the FAP and Internet Samples

of models at the left-hand side of the path diagram. It may also modify your parameter constraints." Click OK, which will bring up a window like that shown in Figure 5.3. The Parameter Subsets set constraints on the models as follows: *(1)* measurement weights constrain the factor loadings to be equal; *(2)* measurement intercepts constrain the "intercepts in the equations for predicted measured variables" (Arbuckle, 2006, p. 384); *(3)* structural weights constrain the regression weights among the latent variables; *(4)* structural intercepts constrain the regression intercept(s) in the model; *(5)* structural means constrain the means of the latent variables; *(6)* structural covariances constrain the variances of the latent variables; *(7)* structural residuals constrain the variance of the structural latent variable; and *(8)* measurement residuals constrain the residuals. Notice in Figure 5.3 that three of the parameter subsets (structural weights, structural intercepts, and structural residuals) are not options for the CFA model to be fitted. This is because the CFA model does not include structural relationships among the latent variables. Also notice that each consecutive model adds additional constrains in a manner similar to that suggested by Brown (2006).

All five models could be fitted to the data, and the model fit summary is shown in Table 5.2. Notice in Table 5.2 that the Model Fit Summary is provided for multiple models. The Unconstrained Model is when the two groups are fitted separately, and there are no equality constraints imposed. Overall, the unconstrained model fits reasonably well, with χ^2 = 369.916, df = 124, χ^2/df = 2.983, TLI = 0.776, CFI = 0.847, RMSEA = 0.092, 90% confidence interval for RMSEA = 0.081 to 0.103, AIC = 537.916, and ECVI = 2.289.

In the Measurement weights model, the measurement weights (i.e., regression coefficients or factor loadings) are constrained to be equal. The Measurement Intercepts are constrained to be equal in the third model; the structural covariances (i.e., the correlations among the latent variables) are constrained in the fourth model; and the measurement residuals (i.e., the errors) are constrained in the fifth model. Notice that

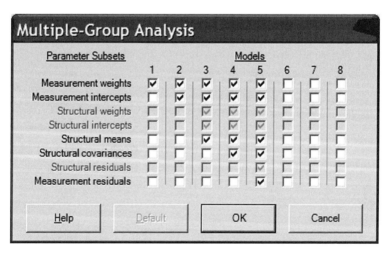

Figure 5.3 Amos 7.0 Graphics Window for Conducting a Multiple-Group Analysis

although χ^2 increases across the five models, the ratio of χ^2/df decreases across the first four models and even in the highly restrictive fifth model, the ratio is still lower than for the unconstrained model. Table 5.3 provides the significance tests for the nested model comparisons. Constraining the measurement weights does not significantly change the model fit ($p = 0.092$) from the unconstrained model. Adding the measurement intercepts constraints results in a significant change from the unconstrained and measurement weights constrained models ($p = 0.001$), but adding the structural covariances does not result in a significant change in model fit from the measurement intercepts constraint model ($p = 0.072$). The TLI and RMSEA both improve slightly as the constraints are added for measurement weights and intercepts and the structural covariances. Although CFI decreases for each model, the decreases are small. Overall,

Table 5.2 Model Fit Summary for the Multiple-Group CFA of the JSS (Amos 7.0 Output)

Model Fit Summary
CMIN

Model	NPAR	CMIN	DF	p	CMIN/DF
Unconstrained	84	369.916	124	0.000	2.983
Measurement weights	74	386.193	134	0.000	2.882
Measurement intercepts	61	421.915	147	0.000	2.870
Structural covariances	55	433.505	153	0.000	2.833
Measurement residuals	42	491.450	166	0.000	2.961
Saturated model	208	0.000	0		
Independence model	26	1790.757	182	0.000	9.839

Baseline Comparisons

Model	NFI Delta1	RFI rho1	IFI Delta2	TLI rho2	CFI
Unconstrained	0.793	0.697	0.852	0.776	0.847
Measurement weights	0.784	0.707	0.848	0.787	0.843
Measurement intercepts	0.764	0.708	0.833	0.788	0.829
Structural covariances	0.758	0.712	0.829	0.793	0.826
Measurement residuals	0.726	0.699	0.800	0.778	0.798
Saturated model	1.000		1.000		1.000
Independence model	0.000	0.000	0.000	0.000	0.000

(*continued*)

Table 5.2 Model Fit Summary for the Multiple-Group CFA of the JSS (Amos 7.0 Output) (*continued*)

Parsimony-Adjusted Measures

Model	p-RATIO	p-NFI	p-CFI
Unconstrained	0.681	0.541	0.577
Measurement weights	0.736	0.577	0.621
Measurement intercepts	0.808	0.617	0.670
Structural covariances	0.841	0.637	0.694
Measurement residuals	0.912	0.662	0.728
Saturated model	0.000	0.000	0.000
Independence model	1.000	0.000	0.000

NCP

Model	NCP	LO 90	HI 90
Unconstrained	245.916	191.962	307.503
Measurement weights	252.193	197.198	314.830
Measurement intercepts	274.915	217.289	340.183
Structural covariances	280.505	222.128	346.527
Measurement residuals	325.450	262.742	395.791
Saturated model	0.000	0.000	0.000
Independence model	1608.757	1476.794	1748.137

FMIN

Model	FMIN	F0	LO 90	HI 90
Unconstrained	1.574	1.046	0.817	1.309
Measurement weights	1.643	1.073	0.839	1.340
Measurement intercepts	1.795	1.170	0.925	1.448
Structural covariances	1.845	1.194	0.945	1.475
Measurement residuals	2.091	1.385	1.118	1.684
Saturated model	0.000	0.000	0.000	0.000
Independence model	7.620	6.846	6.284	7.439

RMSEA

Model	RMSEA	LO 90	HI 90	p-CLOSE
Unconstrained	.092	.081	.103	.000
Measurement weights	.089	.079	.100	.000
Measurement intercepts	.089	.079	.099	.000
Structural covariances	.088	.079	.098	.000
Measurement residuals	.091	.082	.101	.000
Independence model	.194	.186	.202	.000

(*continued*)

Table 5.2 Model Fit Summary for the Multiple-Group CFA of the JSS (Amos 7.0 Output) (*continued*)

AIC

Model	AIC	BCC	BIC	CAIC
Unconstrained	537.916	561.627		
Measurement weights	534.193	555.080		
Measurement intercepts	543.915	561.134		
Structural covariances	543.505	559.030		
Measurement residuals	575.450	587.305		
Saturated model	416.000	474.712		
Independence model	1842.757	1850.096		

ECVI

Model	ECVI	LO 90	HI 90	MECVI
Unconstrained	2.289	2.059	2.551	2.390
Measurement weights	2.273	2.039	2.540	2.362
Measurement intercepts	2.315	2.069	2.592	2.388
Structural covariances	2.313	2.064	2.594	2.379
Measurement residuals	2.449	2.182	2.748	2.499
Saturated model	1.770	1.770	1.770	2.020
Independence model	7.842	7.280	8.435	7.873

HOELTER

Model	HOELTER .05	HOELTER .01
Unconstrained	97	105
Measurement weights	100	108
Measurement intercepts	100	107
Structural covariances	101	108
Measurement residuals	96	103
Independence model	30	32

this pattern of findings suggests that the same JSS model fits the data equally well for the FAP and Internet samples.

Chapter Summary

Multiple-group CFA was presented in this chapter, including considerations for conducting this type of analysis and steps in conducting the analysis. Equality constraints were discussed in detail. Finally, a detailed multiple-group CFA for the JSS was presented.

Table 5.3 Nested Model Comparisons for Multiple Group CFA on the JSS (Amos 7.0 Output)

Nested Model Comparisons
Assuming Model Unconstrained to be Correct:

Model	DF	CMIN	p	NFI Delta-1	IFI Delta-2	RFI rho-1	TLI rho2
Measurement weights	10	16.276	0.092	0.009	0.010	−0.010	−0.011
Measurement intercepts	23	51.999	0.001	0.029	0.031	−0.011	−0.013
Structural covariances	29	63.589	0.000	0.036	0.038	−0.015	−0.017
Measurement residuals	42	121.534	0.000	0.068	0.073	−0.002	−0.003

Assuming Model Measurement Weights to be Correct:

Model	DF	CMIN	p	NFI Delta-1	IFI Delta-2	RFI rho-1	TLI rho2
Measurement intercepts	13	35.723	0.001	0.020	0.022	−0.001	−0.001
Structural covariances	19	47.313	0.000	0.026	0.029	−0.005	−0.006
Measurement residuals	32	105.257	0.000	0.059	0.064	0.008	0.009

Assuming Model Measurement Intercepts to be Correct:

Model	DF	CMIN	p	NFI Delta-1	IFI Delta-2	RFI rho-1	TLI rho2
Structural covariances	6	11.590	0.072	0.006	0.007	−0.004	−0.004
Measurement residuals	19	69.535	0.000	0.039	0.042	0.009	0.010

Assuming Model Structural Covariances to be Correct:

Model	DF	CMIN	p	NFI Delta-1	IFI Delta-2	RFI rho-1	TLI rho2
Measurement residuals	13	57.945	0.000	0.032	0.035	0.013	0.014

Suggestions for Further Reading

Byrne (2001a) provides extensive coverage of testing invariance across groups using Amos, including an example with partial measurement invariance. Byrne (2004) provides additional information on conducting multiple-group CFA using Amos Graphics. Brown (2006) and Kline (2005) discuss MIMIC—multiple indicators, multiple causes—models (also known as CFA with covariates) as an alternative approach to examining invariance in multiple groups. MIMIC models are more limited than multiple groups CFA models regarding what they can test, but they have smaller sample size requirements and may be less cumbersome when there are more than two groups in the analysis. Finally, in addition to the social work CFA examples cited in this chapter, Hertzog, Van Alstine, Usala, Hultsch, and Dixon (1990) provide an example of a multiple-group CFA of the CES-D.

6

Other Issues

Presenting Confirmatory Factor Analysis Results

A good article or presentation reporting the results of a confirmatory factor analysis (CFA) will include sufficient information so that the reader can easily understand how the analysis was performed. Whether you are reading or writing articles using CFA, they should include information on:

- Model specification: The conceptual model should be clearly presented, along with the underlying theory or prior research that guided the initial model specification.
- Input data: The sample and type of data should be clearly described and should indicate how data were checked and how problems (e.g., missing data) were addressed.
- Model estimation: Indicate what software (including version number) and estimation method were used.
- Model evaluation, including:

  - Multiple-fit indices should be reported: Some suggestions and guidelines have been presented here, but different journals may have different requirements.

- Localized areas of strain: how were areas of strain identified.
- Parameter estimates (factor loadings, factor and error variances) and their meaning.
- Rationale for respecification: If the model was respecified, provide the rationale for changes made to the model.
- If you have respecified the model, remind the reader that you have moved from model verification to exploration and that further studies will be needed to verify the respecified model.
- Substantive conclusions: what do the findings mean, and what (if any) additional work is needed on the model.

Longitudinal Measurement Invariance

Confirmatory factor analysis can also be used to test whether construct measurement is invariant over time, which is often assumed, but not tested in longitudinal research. If the assumed invariance does not hold over time, then analyses and conclusions about change over time may be misleading. Specifically, researchers may conclude that the underlying construct changes over time when it is actually the measurement of the construct that changes over time. For example, consider the Children's Depression Inventory (CDI), a 27-item self-report scale for depression in children and young adolescents 8 to 14 years of age (Kovacs, 1992, cited in Craighead, Smucker, Craighead, & Ilardi, 1998). In a large sample of children and adolescents, Craighead and colleagues (1998) found similar factor structures on the CDI for the two groups; however, there was a biological dysregulation factor found for adolescents but not children. Although their CFAs were conducted with cross-sectional data, the findings suggest that the factor structure of the CDI may not be invariant over time, and caution is needed in interpreting longitudinal changes on the CDI.

Brown (2006) suggests that measurement invariance over time should be tested before proceeding with structural equation modeling analyses of longitudinal data. Longitudinal measurement invariance can be tested using the multiple-group CFA approach described in the previous chapter, treating each wave or time-point as a separate group (see Brown, 2006 for other ways of testing longitudinal measurement invariance).

Equivalent Models

Equivalent models have different model specifications but fit the data equally well and yield the same predicted covariance matrices within a given data set (Brown, 2006); they are common in research but are generally ignored, although they should be addressed when reporting CFA results (MacCallum & Austin, 2000). MacCallum and Austin (2000) "urge researchers to generate and evaluate the substantive meaningfulness of equivalent models in empirical studies. Ruling out their existence or meaningfulness would strengthen the support of a favored model. More generally, any effort to examine alternative models can provide some protection against confirmation bias [i.e. favoring the proposed model] and bolster support of a favored model" (p. 213).

Multilevel Confirmatory Factor Analysis Models

Often, data have a clustered or nested structure, such as individual students nested within classrooms. With such data structures, there can be individual level effects (i.e., student effects) and there can be group level effects (i.e., classroom effects) that need to be addressed in the data analysis. Multilevel (or hierarchical) linear modeling can be used to test these types of data structures (for a brief introduction to multilevel linear modeling, see Tabachnick & Fidell, 2007). Whereas multilevel CFA models are beyond the scope of this book, it is important to note that such models are possible and should be considered when data have a nested structure.

Chapter Summary

This chapter provides suggestions for critiquing or reporting CFA results in presentations or publications and very briefly introduces several topics that are important in CFA but are beyond the scope of this book to address in detail, including longitudinal measurement invariance, equivalent models, and multilevel models.

Suggestions for Further Reading

Beadnell, Carlisle, Hoppe, Mariano, Wilsdon, Morrison, Wells, Gillmore, and Higa (2007) provide an example of a multilevel CFA for a measure of adolescent friendship closeness. Brown (2006, Table 4.6, pp. 145–146) provides a thorough list of information to report in a CFA study.

Conclusion

As you may have noticed throughout this book, there are a number of places (e.g., sample size requirements) where there is no consensus on recommendations or guidelines for conducting CFA. Compared to many of the data analysis techniques that social workers commonly use, such as regression or analysis of variance, CFA is a relatively new analysis technique and certain aspects of it are still being developed. It is hoped that this short book pocket has provided you with an overview of this analysis, as well as an introduction to some of the issues involved in using CFA. For each topic discussed, I have tried to provide references and suggestions for further reading that represent the current state of the art in this area, but readers are encouraged to continue to look for new and updated information on CFA as they read and use this technique.

Glossary

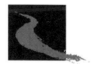

Convergence a set of parameters are estimated that cannot be improved upon to reduce the difference between the predicted and sample covariance matrices

Endogenous variables caused (at least theoretically) by other variables; in this sense they are similar to dependent variables (DV), Y, or outcome variables in regression analyses

Equality constraints parameters are forced to be equal and are not allowed to be freely estimated

Error covariances correlated errors demonstrating that the indicators are related because of something other than the shared influence of the latent factor

Error variance the unique variance in an indicator that is not accounted for by the latent factor(s); also known as measurement error or indicator unreliability

Exogenous variables not caused by other variables in the model; they are similar to an independent variable (IV), X, or predictor in regression analyses

Factor correlation   the relationship between two factors, or latent variables, in the completely standardized solution

Factor covariance   the relationship between two factors, or latent variables, in the unstandardized solution

Factor loadings   the regression coefficients (i.e., slopes) for predicting the indicators from the latent factor

Factor variance   the sample variance for a factor (in the unstandardized solution)

Heywood cases   parameter estimates with out-of-range values

Invariance   equivalence across groups or time

Latent variable   unobserved, unmeasured, underlying construct; usually represented by an oval in CFA or SEM figures

Measurement model   relationships among indicators and latent variables

Method effects   relationships between variables caused by a common measurement method, such as self-reporting

Modification indices   data-driven suggestions available through most software packages about ways to improve the model fit

Observed variable   exactly what it sounds like—a bit of information that is actually observed, such as a person's response to a question or a measured attribute such as weight in pounds; also referred to as indicators or items; usually represented by a rectangle in CFA and SEM figures

Structural model   relationships among latent variables

Appendix A

Brief Introduction to Using Amos

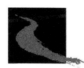

To create the Amos 7.0 Graphics file for running a CFA, click on FILE, then NEW, which will open a blank drawing screen as shown in Figure A.1. The drawing functions in Amos 7.0 are similar to those found in other Windows-based software packages, such as Word and PowerPoint. Icons along the left side of Figure A.1 are used for many of the drawing functions, such as adding observed and latent variables (the rectangle and oval, respectively), adding paths (the left pointing arrow), and adding covariances (the two headed arrow). Resting the cursor on each icon will bring up a small box indicating what it does.

To define the observed and latent variables in the model, right-click on the rectangle or oval, which will bring up a menu of options, including Object Properties. Click on Object Properties. Under Text, you can add variable names and labels, and choose font size and style. "Variable name" must match the variable name in the dataset. Each observed variable must have a "unique variable" or error term, which is indicated by the small circles in the Amos drawing. Error terms can be named anything you wish; in this book they are labeled e and an item number; for instance, in the example presented in Chapter 2, the MBI has 22 items, so the error terms are labeled e1 to e22. The latent variables can be scaled by right-clicking on the regression path for the variable you wish to use to scale each latent variable (e.g., the path from EE to "emotionally drained" in Figure A.2). Right-clicking will bring up a menu of options, including

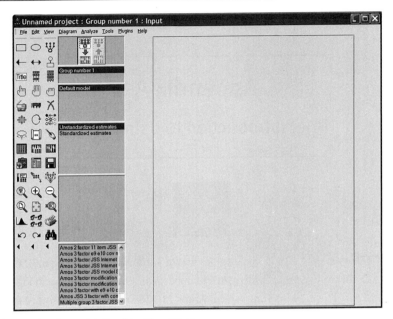

Figure A.1 Amos 7.0 Graphics New File Screen

Object Properties. Click on Object Properties. Under Parameters, you can set the Regression weight to 1 to scale the latent variable. This will create the Amos 7.0 Graphics input file shown in Figure A.2.

Amos 7.0 will read data files from multiple sources. To choose the data for the analysis, click on File, then Data Files, which will bring up the box shown in Figure A.3. Click on File Name, which will allow you to browse through files to find the one you want. After selecting the desired file, click OK. Once the model has been drawn and the appropriate data file opened, you will need to specify the estimation method to be used and the desired output.

To choose the estimation method, click on View, then Analysis Properties, then the Estimation tab, which will bring up the box shown in Figure A.4. Maximum likelihood estimation can be used with complete or incomplete data and is generally the best option as long as the normality assumption is adequately met (this was discussed in detail in Chapter 3).

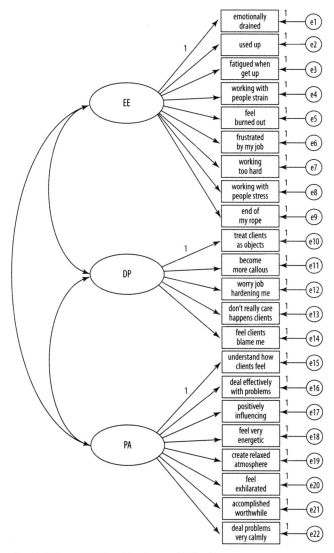

Figure A.2 Amos 7.0 Graphics Input File for the MBI CFA

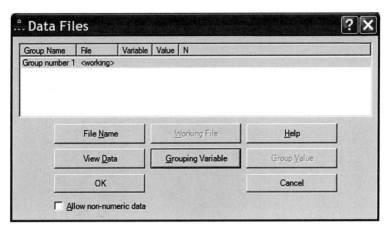

Figure A.3 Amos 7.0 Graphics Data Files Menu

If the data set has missing data, then you must click on Estimate means and intercepts.

To choose the output for the analysis, click on View, then Analysis Properties, then the Output tab, which will bring up the box shown in Figure A.5. Modification indices and Tests for normality and outliers are only available for complete data.

To run the model, click on Analyze, then Calculate Estimates. Then to view all text output, click on View, then Text Output. To view the CFA model with coefficients, click on the "View the output path diagram" and choose Unstandardized estimates or Standardized estimates, as desired. The Standardized output Amos 7.0 Graphics Screen for the MBI example presented in Chapter 2 is shown in Figure A.6. Notice that the Amos 7.0 Graphics screen view shown in Figure A.6 divides the screen into three sections. The left section includes all the icons for many of the commands used in Amos. The middle section (with the darker gray background) provides information on the analysis being conducted. This middle section is divided into six sections, three of which help the user navigate through the output: *(1)* the top section shows two buttons ("view the input path diagram [model specification]" and "view the output path diagram"); these two buttons let you switch back and forth

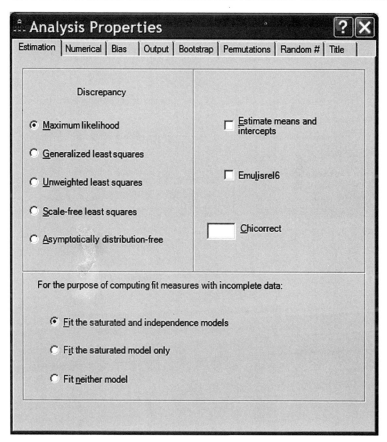

Figure A.4 Amos 7.0 Graphics Analysis Properties Estimation Menu

between viewing the input and output path diagrams; *(2)* the second section identifies the groups used and lets you switch between the output for different groups in a multiple group analysis; and *(3)* the fourth section has "Unstandardized estimates" and "Standardized estimates" and allows you to switch between the two output versions.

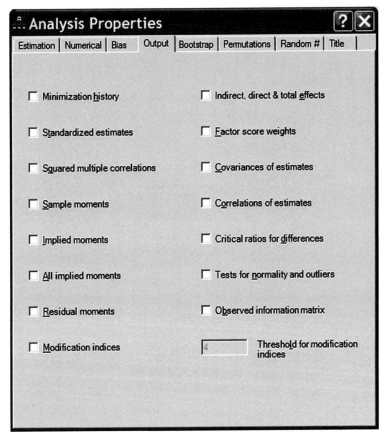

Figure A.5 Amos 7.0 Graphics Analysis Properties Output Menu

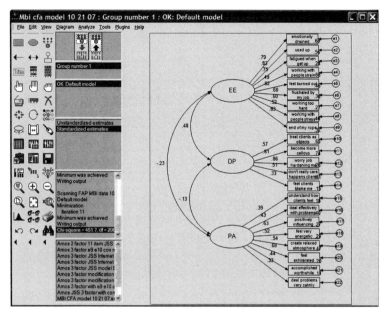

Figure A.6 Standardized Output Screen View in Amos 7.0 Graphics for MBI CFA

References

Abbott, A. A. (2003). A confirmatory factor analysis of the Professional Opinion Scale: A values assessment instrument. *Research on Social Work Practice, 13,* 641–666.

Allison, P. D. (2003). Missing data techniques for structural equation modeling. *Journal of Abnormal Psychology, 112,* 545–557.

Arbuckle, J. L. (2006a). *Amos 7.0.0 (Build 1140).* Spring House, PA: Amos Development Corporation.

Arbuckle, J. L. (2006b). *Amos 7.0 user's guide.* Chicago, IL: SPSS.

Bagozzi, R. P., Yi, Y., & Phillips, L. W. (1991). Assessing construct validity in organizational research. *Administrative Science Quarterly, 36,* 421–458.

Beadnell, B., Carlisle, S. K., Hoppe, M. J., Mariano, K. A., Wilsdon, A., Morrison, D. M., et al. (2007). The reliability and validity of a group-based measure of adolescents' friendship closeness. *Research on Social Work Practice,* doi: 10.1177/1049731506299022.

Bean, N. M., Harrington, D., & Pintello, D. (1998). *Final Report: IASWR/NNF/ UMD/U.S. Air Force FAP Workers Evaluation Project and Post-Doctoral Fellowship.* Baltimore, MD: University of Maryland School of Social Work.

Begun, A. L., Murphy, C., Bolt, D., Weinstein, B., Strodthoff, T., Short, L., et al. (2003). Characteristics of the Safe at Home instrument for assessing readiness to change intimate partner violence. *Research on Social Work Practice, 13,* 80–107.

Belcastro, B. R., & Koeske, G. F. (1996). Job satisfaction and intention to seek graduate education. *Journal of Social Work Education, 32*(3).

Brown, T. A. (2006). *Confirmatory factor analysis for applied research.* New York: The Guilford Press.

Byrne, B. M. (2006). *Structural equation modeling with EQS: Basic concepts, applications, and programming.* Mahwah, NJ: Lawrence Erlbaum Associates, Publishers.

Byrne, B. M. (2004). Testing for multigroup invariance using AMOS Graphics: A road less traveled. *Structural Equation Modeling, 11,* 272–300.

Byrne, B. M. (2001a). *Structural equation modeling with AMOS: Basic concepts, applications, and programming.* Mahwah, NJ: Lawrence Erlbaum Associates, Publishers.

Byrne, B. M. (2001b). Structural equation modeling with AMOS, EQS, and LISREL: Comparative approaches to testing for the factorial validity of a measuring instrument. *International Journal of Testing, 1*(1), 55–86.

Byrne, B. M. (1998). *Structural equation modeling with LISREL, PRELIS, and SIMPLIS: Basic concepts, applications, and programming.* Mahwah, NJ: Lawrence Erlbaum Associates, Publishers.

Chan, Y. C., Lam, G. L. T., Chun, P. K. R., & So, M. T. E. (2006). Confirmatory factor analysis of the Child Abuse Potential Inventory: Results based on a sample of Chinese mothers in Hong Kong. *Child Abuse & Neglect, 30,* 1005–1016. DOI: 10.1016/j.chiabu.2006.05.005.

Cohen, J., Cohen, P., West, S. G., & Aiken, L. S. (2003). *Applied multiple regression/ correlation analysis for the behavioral sciences* (3rd ed.). Mahwah, NJ: Erlbaum.

Craighead, W. E., Smucker, M. R., Craighead, L. W., & Ilardi, S. S. (1998). Factor analysis of the Children's Depression Inventory in a community sample. *Psychological Assessment, 10*(2), 156–165.

Cronbach, L. J., & Meehl, P. E. (1955). Construct validity in psychological tests. *Psychological Bulletin, 52,* 281–302.

Drake, B., & Yadama, G. N. (1995). Confirmatory factor analysis of the Maslach Burnout Inventory. *Social Work Research, 19,* 184–192.

Enders, C. K. (2001). A primer on maximum likelihood algorithms available for use with missing data. *Structural Equation Modeling, 8*(1), 128–141.

Gignac, G. E. (2006). Self-reported emotional intelligence and life satisfaction: Testing incremental predictive validity hypotheses via structural equation modeling (SEM) in a small sample. *Personality and Individual Differences, 40,* 1569–1577.

Gold, M. S., Bentler, P. M., & Kim, K. H. (2003). A comparison of maximum-likelihood and asymptotically distribution-free methods of treating incomplete nonnormal data. *Structural Equation Modeling, 10,* 47–79.

Golob, T. F. (2003). Structural equation modeling for travel behavior research. *Transportation Research Part B, 37,* 1–25.

Graham, J. W. (2003). Adding missing-data-relevant variables to FIML-based structural equation models. *Structural Equation Modeling, 10*(1), 80–100.

Grimm, L. G., & Yarnold, P. R. (2000). *Reading and understanding more multivariate statistics.* Washington, DC: American Psychological Association.

Grimm, L. G., & Yarnold, P. R. (1994). *Reading and understanding multivariate statistics.* Washington, D.C: American Psychological Association.

Greeno, E. J., Hughes, A. K., Hayward, R. A., & Parker, K. L. (2007). A confirmatory factor analysis of the Professional Opinion Scale. *Research on Social Work Practice, 17,* 482–493.

Haig, B. D. (2005). Exploratory factor analysis, theory generation, and scientific method. *Multivariate Behavioral Research, 40,* 303–329.

Harrington, D., Bean, N., Pintello, D., & Mathews, D. (2001). Job satisfaction and burnout: Predictors of intentions to leave a job in a military setting. *Administration in Social Work, 25*(3), 1–16.

Harrington, D., Zuravin, S., DePanfilis, D., Ting, L., & Dubowitz, H. (2002). The Neglect Scale: Confirmatory factor analysis in a low-income sample. *Child Maltreatment, 7,* 259–368.

Haynes, S. N., Richard, D. C. S., & Kubany, E. S. (1995). Content validity in psychological assessment: A functional approach to concepts and methods. *Psychological Assessment, 7,* 238–247.

Hays, R. D., Revicki, D., & Coyne, K. S. (2005). Application of structural equation modeling to health outcomes research. *Evaluation & the Health Professions, 28,* 295–309.

Hertzog, C., Van Alstine, J., Usala, P. D., Hultsch, D. F., & Dixon, R. (1990). Measurement properties of the Center for Epidemiological Studies Depression Scale (CES-D) in older populations. *Psychological Assessment: A Journal of Consulting and Clinical Psychology, 2,* 64–72.

Jöreskog, K., & Sörbom, D. (2006). *LISREL 8.80* (July 2006). Lincolnwood, IL: Scientific Software International.

Jöreskog, K., & Sörbom, D. (2006). *PRELIS 2.80* (2006). Lincolnwood, IL: Scientific Software International.

Kline, R. B. (2005). *Principles and practice of structural equation modeling* (2nd ed.). New York: The Guilford Press.

Koeske, G. F. (1994). Some recommendations for improving measurement validation in social work research. *Journal of Social Service Research, 18*(3/4), 43–72.

Koeske, G. F., Kirk, S. A., Koeske, R. D., & Rauktis, M. E. (1994). Measuring the Monday blues: Validation of a job satisfaction scale for the human services. *Social Work Research, 18,* 27–35.

Koeske, G. F., & Kelly, T. (1995). The impact of overinvolvement on burnout and job satisfaction. *American Journal of Orthopsychiatry, 65,* 282–292.

Lee, S.-Y., & Song, X.-Y. (2004). Evaluation of the Bayesian and maximum likelihood approaches in analyzing structural equation models with small sample sizes. *Multivariate Behavioral Research, 39,* 653–686.

Long, J. S. (1983). *Confirmatory factor analysis: A preface to LISREL* (Sage University Paper series on Quantitative Applications in the Social Sciences, No. 07–033). Newbury Park, CA: Sage.

MacCallum, R. C. (2003). Working with imperfect models. *Multivariate Behavioral Research, 38*(1), 113–139.

MacCallum, R. C., & Austin, J. T. (2000). Applications of structural equation modeling in psychological research. *Annual Review of Psychology, 51,* 201–226.

MacCallum, R. C., Browne, M. W., & Sugawara, H. M. (1996). Power analysis and determination of sample size for covariance structure modeling. *Psychological Methods, 1,* 130–149.

MacCallum, R. C., & Hong, S. (1997). Power analysis in covariance structure modeling using GFI and AGFI. *Multivariate Behavioral Research, 32,* 193–210.

MacCallum, R. C., Widaman, K. F., Preacher, K. J., & Hong, S. (2001). Sample size in factor analysis: The role of model error. *Multivariate Behavioral Research, 36,* 611–637.

Macgowan, M. J., & Newman, F. L. (2005). Factor structure of the Group Engagement Measure. *Social Work Research, 29,* 107–118.

Maslach, C., Jackson, S. E., & Leiter (1996). *Maslach Burnout Inventory* (3rd ed.). Palo Alto, CA: Consulting Psychologists Press, Inc.

Meyers, L. S., Gamst, G., & Guarino, A. J. (2006). *Applied multivariate research: Design and interpretation.* Thousand Oaks: Sage Publications.

Muthén, L. K., & Muthén, B. O. (2002). How to use a Monte Carlo study to decide on sample size and determine power. *Structural Equation Modeling, 9,* 599–620.

Preacher, K. J., & MacCallum, R. C. (2002). Exploratory factor analysis in behavior genetics research: Factor recovery in small sample sizes. *Behavior Genetics, 32,* 153–161.

Podsakoff, P. M., MacKenzie, S. B., Lee, J.-Y., & Podsakoff, N. P. (2003). Common method biases in behavioral research: A critical review of the literature and recommended remedies. *Journal of Applied Psychology, 88,* 879–903.

Radloff, L. S. (1977). The CES-D scale: A self-report depression scale for research in the general population. *Applied Psychological Measurement, 1,* 385–401.

Raykov, T., & Marcoulides, G. A. (2006). *A first course in structural equation modeling* (2nd ed.). Mahwah, NJ: Lawrence Erlbaum Associates, Inc.

Raykov, T., Tomer, A., & Nesselroade, J. R. (1991). Reporting structural equation modeling results in *Psychology and Aging:* Some proposed guidelines. *Psychology and Aging, 6,* 499–503.

Reilly, T. (1995). A necessary and sufficient condition for identification of confirmatory factor analysis models of factor complexity one. *Sociological Methods & Research, 23,* 421–441.

Saris, W. E., & Satorra, A. (1993). Power evaluations in structural equation models. In K. A. Bollen & J. S. Long (Eds.), *Testing structural equation models* (pp. 181–204). Newbury Park, CA: Sage.

Satorra, A., & Saris, W. E. (1985). Power of the likelihood ratio test in covariance structure analysis. *Psychometrika, 50,* 83–90.

Savalei, V., & Bentler, P. M. (2005). A statistically justified pairwise ML method for incomplete nonnormal data: A comparison with direct ML and pairwise ADF. *Structural Equation Modeling, 12,* 183–214.

Schafer, J. L., & Graham, J. W. (2002). Missing data: Our view of the state of the art. *Psychological Methods, 7,* 147–177.

Schaufeli, W., & Van Dierendonck, D. (1995). A cautionary note about the cross-national and clinical validity of cut-off points for the Maslach Burnout Inventory. *Psychological Reports, 76,* 1083–1090.

Shadish, W. R., Cook, T. D., & Campbell, D. T. (2002). *Experimental and quasi-experimental designs for generalized causal inference.* New York: Houghton Mifflin Company.

Shete, S., Beasley, T. M., Etzel, C. J., Fernández, J. R., Chen, J., Allison, D. B., et al. (2004). Effect of winsorization on power and type I error of variance components and related methods of QTL detection. *Behavior Genetics, 34*(2), 153–159.

Siebert, D. C., & Siebert, C. F. (2005). The Caregiver Role Identity Scale: A validation study. *Research on Social Work Practice, 15,* 204–212. DOI: 10.1177.1049731504272779.

SPSS, Inc. (2006). *SPSS for Windows 15.0.* www.spss.com (accessed on 9 June 2008).

Stevens, J. P. (2002). *Applied multivariate statistics for the social sciences* (4th ed.). Mahwah, NJ: Lawrence Erlbaum Associates.

Straus, M. A., Kinard, E. M., & Williams, L. M. (1995, July 23). *The Neglect Scale.* Paper presented at the Fourth International Conference on Family Violence Research, Durham, NH.

Tabachnick, B. G., & Fidell, L. S. (2007). *Using multivariate statistics* (5th ed.). Boston: Allyn and Bacon.

Thompson, B. (2004). *Exploratory and confirmatory factor analysis: Understanding concepts and applications.* Washington, D.C: APA Books.

van Saane, N., Sluiter, J. K., Verbeek, J. H. A. M., & Frings-Dresen, M. H. W. (2003). Reliability and validity of instruments measuring job satisfaction—a systematic review. *Occupational Medicine, 53,* 191–200.

Yuan, K.-H., & Bentler, P. M. (2001). Effect of outliers on estimators and tests in covariance structure analysis. *British Journal of Mathematical and Statistical Psychology, 54,* 161–175.

Yuan, K.-H., & Bentler, P. M. (2004). On chi-square difference and z tests in mean and covariance structure analysis when the base model is misspecified. *Educational and Psychological Measurement, 64,* 737–757.

Yuan, K.-H., Bentler, P. M., & Zhang, W. (2005). The effect of skewness and kurtosis on mean and covariance structure analysis: The univariate case and its multivariate implication. *Sociological Methods & Research, 34,* 240–258.

Index

Amos 7.0, 3, 12, 13, 28–31, 92, 94,
    107–113
Asymptotically distribution free
    (ADF), 29, 30, 35, 45

Categorical data, 29, 30, 36, 44, 45, 46
Common factor model, 9, 10, 11
Congeneric indicators, 82
Content validity, 20
Continuous data, 29, 31, 32, 44, 45
Construct validity, 5–7, 15, 17, 20
Convergent validity, 6–7
Criterion validity, 6

Data considerations, 36–49, 59, 79–80
Default model, 66
Discriminant validity, 6–7, 18

Endogenous variable, 23, 105
Equality constraint, 46, 79, 81–82,
    92, 105
Equivalent models, 102
Error covariance, 24, 27, 54, 81, 105

Error variance, 24, 27, 29, 82, 105
Exogenous variable, 23, 105
Exploratory factor analysis (EFA), 4,
    9–10, 11, 47

Factor correlation, 24, 106
Factor covariance, 24, 81, 106
Factor loading, 22, 23, 24, 27, 46, 53,
    62, 63, 78, 81, 82, 93, 94, 106
Factor variance, 24, 27, 78, 81, 106
Factorial validity (see structural validity)
Fit indices, 50–52

Generalized least squares (GLS)
    estimation, 28, 30
Goodness of fit (GFI) index, 41, 47

Heywood case, 29, 43, 106

Identification, 21, 24–27
Imputation, 30, 39–41
Indicator variable (see observed
    variable)

Independence model, 66
Indicator unreliability (see error variance)

Just-identified model, 25

Kurtosis, 30, 41–45, 48, 61, 68–69

Latent variable, 5, 7, 9–12, 22, 23, 25–26, 54, 62–63, 75, 78–79, 81–83, 93–94, 107–108
Longitudinal invariance, 101

Maximum likelihood (ML) estimation, 28–30, 40–41, 44–46, 48
Measurement development, 4, 5, 21
Measurement error (see error variance)
Measurement invariance, 3, 8, 79–81
Measurement model, 11–12, 27, 78–79, 106
Method effects, 7–8, 24, 106
Missing at random (MAR), 37, 40
Missing completely at random (MCAR), 37, 39, 40
Missing data, 30, 36–41, 46, 48, 59, 61, 110
Model evaluation (see model fit)
Model fit, 52–53
Model revision, 53–56
Model specification, 21–24
Modification indices (MI), 54, 68, 70
Multilevel CFA, 102
Multiple group CFA, 8, 78–99, 101, 111

Nested data, 102
Nested models, 51, 52, 55–56, 71, 81, 82, 95
Normality, 41–42
Nomological validity (see theoretical validity)

Nonignorable missing data, 37–38, 41

Observed variable, 9, 22, 23, 62, 82, 106
Ordinal data, 29, 44, 45
Outliers, 41, 42–43, 110
Over-identified model, 25–26

Parallel indicators, 82
Parameters, 22, 23–24
Parent model, 55
Principal components analysis (PCA), 9, 10–11

Regression coefficient, 22, 23, 94, 106
Reliability, 4, 7, 24, 46, 63

Sample size requirements, 29, 30, 31, 45–48
Saturated model, 66
Scaling latent variables, 26
Shared method (see method effects)
Skewness, 42, 43, 45, 48, 68
Structural equation modeling (SEM), 9, 11–12, 62
Structural model, 11, 78, 106
Structural validity, 7, 17

Tau-equivalent models, 82
Theoretical validity, 6
Theory, 5, 10, 21–22, 48, 53, 54

Under-identified model, 25
Unweighted least squares (ULS) estimation, 28, 29, 30

Validity, 5–7

Weighted least squares (WLS) estimation, 28, 29, 30